Teaching the Alexander Technique

of related interest

Galvanizing Performance
The Alexander Technique as a Catalyst for Excellence
Edited by Cathy Madden and Kathleen Juhl
ISBN 978 1 78592 720 1
eISBN 978 0 85701 272 2

Principles of the Alexander Technique
What It is, How It Works, and What It Can Do for You
Second Edition
Jeremy Chance
ISBN 978 1 84819 128 0
eISBN 978 0 85701 105 3

Awakening Somatic Intelligence
Understanding, Learning and Practicing the Alexander
Technique, Feldenkrais Method and Hatha Yoga
Graeme Lynn
ISBN 978 1 84819 334 5
eISBN 978 0 85701 290 6

Using Expressive Arts to Work with Mind, Body and Emotions
Theory and Practice
Mark Pearson and Helen Wilson
ISBN 978 1 84905 031 9
eISBN 978 0 85700 189 4

TEACHING THE ALEXANDER TECHNIQUE

Active Pathways to Integrative Practice

CATHY MADDEN

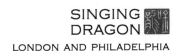

SINGING
DRAGON
LONDON AND PHILADELPHIA

First published in 2018
by Singing Dragon, an imprint of
Jessica Kingsley Publishers
73 Collier Street
London N1 9BE, UK
and
400 Market Street, Suite 400
Philadelphia, PA 19106, USA

www.singingdragon.com

Copyright © Cathy Madden 2018

Front cover image source: Debra Rozin, MD.

Library of Congress Cataloging in Publication Data
A CIP catalog record for this book is available from the Library of Congress

British Library Cataloguing in Publication Data
A CIP catalogue record for this book is available from the British Library

ISBN 978 1 84819 388 8
eISBN 978 0 85701 346 0

Printed and bound in Great Britain

To Alyssa-Lois, Edan-Hoelan, and Steve,
whose choice to say "yes" to themselves, each other,
and the world inspires and delights me

Cherishing the memory of
Lois H. and Stephen F. Madden
and
Marjorie Barstow

Acknowledgments

Everyone I have taught has contributed to what is written in this book. I expect the people I am teaching now and future students will create the next revisions and the new stories to come. As I write this, flashes of our work together are with me.

The students of my Seattle studio, many of whom are the storytellers within the text, many of whom have become teachers of this work via the Living Room Étude. All of whom have advanced my work.

The University of Washington School of Drama—my colleagues, past and present, the alumni and current students of our Professional Actor Training Program, and the BAs who have had the opportunity to study with me.

All my teachers, especially Marjorie Barstow, whose daily diligence in their classrooms set the bar high for me as I walk the path of this profession.

Ken Anno for the initial visualization of my teaching plan; Alyssa-Lois Madden Gehman for its new graphic representation.

My family.

Matt Goodrich for expansive editorial expertise. Through his open-handedness and astute questioning, the words have become a musical composition, moving you in a dance from idea to idea. And Skooter.

Jessica Kingsley and her staff, particularly acknowledging Samantha Patrick and Victoria Peters, for their deep consideration of this topic and care-full ushering of this book to publication.

Contents

Part Three: Integrative Teaching Practice

Introduction

"How did you think of that?" is the question I am most often asked when I am teaching. Each time I am asked, I answer it as completely as I can. And, however I answer, there is a subterranean pastiche of experience and skills and beliefs that created the idea appearing at that moment in time. As with talking about anything and everything Alexander Technique-related, I wish for a tongue that could say many things at once when asked to explain where an idea came from. These writings collect the influences, skills, and experimentation that create the act, perhaps the art, of teaching the Alexander Technique.

The movement through the book begins with acknowledging, in Part One, the background and training shaping my perspective on the Alexander Technique. Part Two of the book considers the essential skills in teaching, with Teaching Stories contributed by students and colleagues offering examples of specific lessons. In Part Three, I offer theoretical background related to my teaching practice, including acting training, studies in adult education (andragogy), and research on human performance and creativity, as well as input from everyone who has ever studied with me. Initially, these theories helped me explain what I was already doing; now, knowing them, they further develop my skills. This part moves into practical application of the accumulated skill sets and ideas in a wide variety of teaching situations. A glimpse into a myriad of games possibilities and a variety of teaching tips provide resources. I close with wishes on the future of teaching this work.

My hope is that the whole book is both a teaching text and teaching resource. While there is a logic to its sequence of chapters, you could drop into any chapter if there is something specific you need or are interested in. (You might need to check in on the Cathy

Glossary in Chapter 2 if you drop into the middle of the book, as I have a propensity to make up words and terms.)

The references offered within the text aim to acknowledge the many fields that contribute to evolving the understanding and teaching of the Alexander Technique. While the book is intended for people who are teaching the Alexander Technique, the truth is that, ultimately, all of us must teach ourselves this elegant process. For anyone reading this as a student of the Alexander Technique, the ideas in this book offer you an opportunity to take on that role of teacher for yourself.

My hope is that each person who reads this is inspired to think of the stories and ideas that they would add to each of the chapters. Each of us is ultimately the evolutioner of our own development.

Part One

MY JOURNEY TO TEACHING THE ALEXANDER TECHNIQUE

Chapter 1

MARJ'S LIVING ROOM

Walking on a beach in Maine with a friend, I mentioned something about being an Alexander Technique teacher; he gently, kindly contradicted me: "You are a teacher. The Alexander Technique is the practice guiding your teaching." This is the spirit and perspective that animates this book—commencing with acknowledging my source and inspiration, my Alexander Technique teacher-mentor Marjorie Barstow (1899–1994, hereafter referred to as Marj).

While I was working on my Master's degree in Theatre at Washington University in St. Louis, Professor of Theatre Sid Friedman invited Marj to give a workshop. He had studied with her at a summer theatre movement workshop and told me, "I think you'd like it." In the acting studio at Edison Theatre, Marj introduced the Alexander Technique to a circle of 20 or so university students. What I remember from that first day was how she moved, talked, taught—and piqued my curiosity. I was particularly fascinated by the increase in theatrical presence I experienced in watching my fellow actors. As we had shared classes for a year, I was familiar with their movement and sound. Something happened in these lessons, however, that invited me to be with them in a way I hadn't experienced before. Fortunately, Sid invited Marj to the university multiple times over the course of my program.

I knew Marj was considered one of the best Alexander Technique teachers in the world, had studied with F.M. Alexander himself, and lived in Lincoln, Nebraska. From Sid, I learned that people learned to teach the work through studying with her. This was the entirety of my research about Alexander Technique teacher training. I wrote Marj a letter saying that I would like to move to Lincoln and learn how to teach with her. "Would that be okay?" I received a note back (how I wish I had kept it!): "Why don't you come along and see what happens?" And so I moved to Nebraska.

At the time, Marj taught two large workshops per year (summer and winter) and held classes twice weekly at her house, usually from 5:30 to 7:30 p.m. I attended as often as I could, all the while acting, directing, and working a day job. These classes formed the foundation of my learning. The format for these workshops and classes was primarily turn-based; that is, if you had something you wanted to do, you raised your hand and asked for a turn. Walking, singing, reaching for things, dancing, running, sewing—anything you wanted to explore.

Living Room Étude

What follows is a description of the journey by which I became the teacher I am today. This is also the core of how I choose to teach people to teach.

Marj did not treat learning to teach any differently than experimenting with your walking. Teaching was just another activity, and if you wanted to learn to do it, you asked to teach for your turn in class. The first time I ventured "I would like to teach" was a benchmark moment. I wish I could say that I specifically remember raising my voice to take this step. I don't. What I do remember are the many times I had wanted to say this and didn't. Believing that I had developed enough skills to take on this task took me quite a while. One day, my desire to learn to teach became stronger than my fear of failure.

> *The act of learning to teach begins with your volition, your desire. Marj didn't "care" if you taught, and she would happily provide you with the tools you needed–if* **you wanted to teach.**

Any time I asked to teach, the atmosphere in the room shifted. Marj sat down and looked expectantly in my direction—turning the teaching space over to me.

> *If you asked to teach for your turn, Marj, by sitting down, was telling you that you were now taking full responsibility for your own coordination.*

My first job was to find someone who wanted to be my student.

In taking on this task, you changed your role, your relationship to the people in the room, and your responsibility to the people in the room. No "in between" existed–no "sort of" or "practice" teaching–you were now the teacher.

Next, as I intended to start the lesson, Marj would ask, "What do you notice about yourself?" When I could answer this question clearly, using what I knew to address any concerns constructively, she invited me to resume. If I got stuck in some way, she'd say, "Why don't you think about that for a while?"

What potent messages she put in this simple, elegant learning experience! As a teacher, your ability to coordinate is your own responsibility. Your job is to think–to analyze and solve your own dilemmas. She didn't help you get unstuck, but, rather, offered the respect of knowing that you could figure it out for yourself. She often reminded us, "The teacher is the most important person in the lesson," and your first job was to be using the Alexander Technique yourself. Questions about the student came next, but only after you were fully using what you knew in service of your own coordination.

As I learned to teach, I realized that *notice* was anything that comes to one's attention. If I happened to receive sensory feedback about my coordination, that was part of the information she was guiding me to use, but such feedback wasn't required. It became apparent that what was vital was what I was thinking as well as the relationship of these thoughts to the accomplishment of my intentions.

As my teaching turn began, I would start to roll forward over my hip joint to stand and walk to my student. Inevitably, just as I barely began to move, Marj would ask, "What do you notice about yourself?" Based on my current experience, I am fairly certain that she asked the question because she had seen that something in my use of myself had gone awry. My job was to respond to her question clearly, then use my "noticing" to reinitiate using the Alexander Technique. Many times, my lesson in teaching ended before I even started to move or talk to my student.

When I responded constructively, Marj introduced a second question: "What do you notice about your student?"

We needed to be able to say in words what we observed and heard (what I would now call "omniservation"). In this practice, I learned

to experience my student as a whole individual and to describe
what I saw accurately and nonjudgmentally.

If I could answer this question clearly, I could go on. If not, I heard:
"Why don't you think about that for a while?"

Many, many months of the same questions:

"What do you notice about yourself?"

"What do you notice about your student?"

Some of my turns lasted less than a minute before, "Why don't you think about that for a while?" Others continued for a bit longer. Perhaps nine months passed before I actually got close enough to my student to use my hands as part of the teaching process. And, because I was constructively coordinating to my task and had developed the necessary skills over the full course of my study, using my hands to teach was immediately a clear and easy event. This success was made possible because of the rigor of the repeating "What do you notice?" practice combined with the skills I was developing in other ways.

Everything You Do Is About Learning to Teach

Responding to Marj's delicate, insistent challenges in the Living Room Étude required a robust, resilient skill set. Indeed, every experiment I had or observed other people having with her facilitated my teaching. Her words still ring: "Every lesson you have is about learning to teach."

While instructing, Alexander Technique teachers walk, talk, think, reach, receive, process, analyze sensory input, puzzle, formulate questions, imitate the student, laugh, look at books, and do many other things. All of these activities were part and parcel of the classes and workshops Marj taught. I applied F.M. Alexander's process repeatedly to those tasks and others. Each experiment refined my ability and overall understanding. I became more constructive, more efficient, more diligent at using what I knew in more situations. I was integrating knowledge and behavior in the service of desire.

These pursuits of daily life—which I examined in virtually every Marj lesson, then studied, analyzed, and practiced, practiced, practiced—contribute to the moment of teaching. They aren't set ideas; rather, they are processes designed to evolve constructively, continually, and forever. The name I have coined for these ever-evolving components is *studied rehearsed plans.*

Studied Rehearsed Plans

Studied rehearsed plans are developed skills that serve the desired action. In using the Alexander Technique to do something, the first part of the rehearsed plan summons the underlying coordination: "Ask myself to COORDINATE so that my head can move so that all of me can follow so that I can do what I am doing" with "what I am doing" as the subsequent part of the plan—the instructions specific to my activity. At this moment of writing, I am asking myself to COORDINATE so that my head can move so that all of me can follow so that I can continue to move in my kneeling chair as I think and move my fingers to the appropriate keys on the keyboard.

Impressions

As workshops concluded, Marj asked participants to write their impressions. This gave us an opportunity to reflect on what had happened during the previous weeks. And she read them to further her own understanding of teaching. Following are my impressions of how the Living Room Étude guides my approach to teaching. With these seven impressions, I offer a context for the ensuing chapters about teaching:

1. I Want to Teach!

2. Responsibility and Confidence

3. Relationship/Communication

4. "Minking" and "Thoving"

5. Omniservation

6. Constructive Thinking

7. Rediscovery of *The Use of the Self*

While I expound on all of these ideas throughout the book, their presentation here is specific to my reflections on learning them from Marj. I imagine she would enjoy knowing that these are the seeds enabling me to continually recreate my own process as my understanding and experience of them deepens. She insisted that we each teach in our own way.

Impression One: I Want to Teach!

The importance of *my* desire as the root of *my* learning is something I understood many years after Marj created the conditions in which I would embrace my freedom of choice in learning. I articulated it for myself for the first time in August 1994, in the first month after Marj died. Her funeral was to take place while I was teaching in Europe. I considered canceling the trip, but when I asked myself the question "Would Marj want me to teach or come to her funeral?" the answer was clear—go teach!

I planned to sit on the balcony of a hotel in the Voralps in Switzerland during the time of the funeral. I hoped for a candle. As I entered the only tiny shop in the small mountain village, I saw every nook and cranny miraculously and mysteriously stuffed with goods. A woman who looked like an ancient granny greeted me in Swiss German and (I imagine) asked me what I wanted. I didn't know the word for *candle*, so I drew a picture. She disappeared into the back of the shop for a few minutes and emerged carrying a small candle. With the grace of this acquisition, I sat on the balcony as the sun set, joining the funeral from afar.

Following my mountain retreat, I was teaching a residential workshop. Most of the participants were Alexander Technique teachers. Following so soon after Marj's death, many questions were about her and my training with her. One question in particular provoked my attention: "Marj teachers are different. What makes them different?"

At this point in my career, I had taught at a variety of Alexander Technique teacher training courses where people were learning to teach in ways different than my experience. As I considered how to answer the question, it occurred to me that the most important difference between what I saw in training schools and heard from people who had learned to teach through that route is the "I want"—desire. Marj had class at various times—she unlocked her front door and whoever wanted to come appeared. We never "had" to come. Everything was volitional.

The Living Room Étude required me to say, "I want to teach"—every time. I can't remember Marj ever saying, "Now, let's work on your teaching." She taught this "Ask for what you want" ethos continuously. Every class and workshop was facilitated with "Who wants to do something?" If you wanted a turn, you asked. And in a large group class, you got great practice in pursuing your desire to express what you needed and wanted. If you didn't find a way to ask, you probably didn't get a turn. Every class I took enabled me to strengthen my studied rehearsed plan for coordinating so that I could express what I wanted.

Reminders of our freedom to choose were abundant in all of our classes and lessons. Marj's invitation "Everybody have a good slump!" was one of many playful reminders of the importance of desire. Being a particular way was not the stated goal. Rather, the freedom to *choose* how you wanted to be was celebrated and insisted upon!

Impression Two: Responsibility and Confidence

I overheard someone who learned to teach with me telling a newer student that when he started to learn to teach, he was a bit shocked—I think he said I turned into a bit of a bear (or was it a dragon?). I laughed because he was articulating clearly a big change that happens when someone asks to teach. I experienced this alteration in Marj as well—suddenly, she seemed to offer me no help at all! In the conversation I eavesdropped upon, my student articulated how much he—like me—ultimately valued this sudden "dragonlike" shift in the teaching relationship.

Why the big change? Teaching involves responsibility. When I declared, "I want to teach," I became responsible for my own coordination while in relationship with another person or people. I was saying that I was ready to be "response-able": able to respond to create the conditions in which they could learn.

I remember that, often, when I or another said, "I want to teach," Marj would sit. At the time, I didn't understand what a clear, powerful, respectful message she was giving. Yet, with that simple move, she acknowledged my belief that I was ready to teach. She held me to a high standard of performance, rooted in my belief in my own skill and expertise.

When I behaved in a way that did not match this standard, I needed to "think about it for a while." Again, in retrospect, I understand the importance of the "think about it for a while" moment. Marj did not solve my dilemma. She entrusted me with the analysis and solution—respecting my belief that I had the skills to reason these out for myself. A great benefit was that this would also develop my ability to analyze the information proffered by my students, letting their input dance with my knowledge and experience to synthesize a doable action plan moving them toward their desire.

As I was held to the standards of my own belief in myself and—over time—succeeded, I became confident in my ability to respond to the needs within lessons, classes, and workshops. Response-ability begot confidence, and both are deeply integrated in my approach to teaching.

Marj alluded to what she expected of teachers as she taught. Periodically, she would ask the group, "Who's the most important person in the lesson?" In call-and-response fashion, we learned to chorus, "The teacher!" The genuine, rigorous, constructive commitment to self that is at the heart of the Alexander Technique is the very foundation for teaching the work. In a moment with Marj in her study—dolls from her vast collection peering down from their perches on top of stuffed bookcases—she said to me, "The Alexander Technique requires the greatest honesty of anything I have ever studied." For me, such honesty began in Marj's living room.

Impression Three: Relationship/Communication

Invisibly, the Living Room Étude taught the basic skills of communication. Moreover, my study of the Alexander Technique was from the beginning communication-centered, because my inquiries were often acting- and performance-based.

The consistent practice of coordinating in the presence of another person, as the Living Room Étude requires—simply to be with them as they were choosing (as my student) to be with me—set up what psychologists call a "relational field." With the aid of the Alexander Technique, this presence becomes a coordination-enhanced field. In theatre, such a field encompasses both the performer-to-performer and performer-to-audience relationships. What we were practicing with Marj was a conscious constructive approach to communication, with clear teacher-to-student relationships creating an enhanced interactive field each time we entered the Living Room Étude.

Marj was widely known as a master communicator. At one point, some Neuro-Linguistic Programming (NLP) specialists came to a workshop particularly to watch her because they had heard how well she communicated. Although she seldom directly addressed communication (though she did ban mumbling), I know I learned osmotically from being in her teaching arena as much as I could. In the Living Room Étude, her coaching was simple: "Don't just look at them, talk to them."

Impression Four: "Minking" and "Thoving"

As I teach, I walk, I talk, I listen, I reach for things, and so forth. All of these activities and other teaching components correspond to the studied rehearsed plans referred to earlier. Lessons on everyday activities and events—both my own and others'—fed my ability to teach, by building the detailed skills that make up these studied rehearsed plans.

I coined the words *minking* and *thoving* when a particular student so strongly separated thought and movement that saying either word became unproductive. Instead, we switched the initial sounds of the words to make "minking" and "thoving." Although Marj didn't use these words, they emphasize the wholeness inherent in how she taught me to teach. In F.M. Alexander language, this is psychophysical unity. The medical field uses the term *biopsychosocial*, and I have recently taken to adopting this term in my practice.

The skills of using your hands and touch as part of the teaching process was something that I and my colleagues knew we needed, but it seemed at least at first a bit mysterious. When we asked about this, Marj said, "If you want to know about using your hands in teaching, watch how you use them all day." Those of us who were learning to teach devised various activities reaching for objects and doing myriad other things with our hands. She instructed us in these activities using words that she also used in relationship to teaching:

"Let your fingers lead to the object."

"Look at your hand as you reach for the object."

"Let the object shape your hand."

I would now word this: "Look at your hand as you lead with your fingers to reach for the object in such a way that your hand moves along the shape of the object."

Marj often remarked that if you are looking at your hands and see that you stiffen, you could use this information to make a new choice. Furthermore, when you watch your hands as they move toward an object, you also see what you are reaching for, which in teaching is your student. If you make contact with the object in such a way that the object shapes your hand, you are discovering it, responding to its details. That is, rather than having a preconceived idea about the object, you discover it as you touch it. The implications of this practice in relationship to using my hands as part of my teaching process are profound. I believe that how I learned to reach for things, and eventually for people, fosters respect for each student. I intend to be with them, meet them where they are, and follow them as they experiment with new ideas.

One day, I decided to take Marj's "Watch what you do with your hands all day" seriously. I even remember doing whole dances involving using the Alexander Technique while I watched my hands in movement. I enjoyed watching my hands as I picked up my children, intending to disturb their coordination as little as possible. Reaching for everything became inherently enjoyable. Integrating using my hands this way all day was my ultimate minking and thoving practice. The many repetitions of the "how" for reaching and touching became my foundational studied rehearsed plan for using my hands while doing anything, including teaching.

Impression Five: Omniservation

Omniservation—another word I coined but believe that Marj taught— is a skill that was cultivated from day one of learning with her. How my classmates changed while Marj taught them was one of my biggest initial impressions of the Alexander Technique. Although I can't remember what Marj actually said to introduce the work, I do know that in my accumulated experience of her work, she asked people to see—and talk about what they saw—right away:

"What do you see?"

"What do you notice?"

These questions were directed not only to the student who had just had a learning moment, but also to everyone in the room. Almost every lesson! If you watch any videos of Marj teaching, you hear these queries often.

When I first studied with Marj, I didn't see much. Hearing the question so frequently, however, indicated that seeing something was possible. Because I mostly studied with groups representing a wide range of experience with the Alexander Technique, someone else might answer the question, giving me an idea of what to look for. Sometimes, the person having a turn would describe what they noticed in themselves, and this also guided my process of learning to omniserve. Other times, I'd say that I hadn't seen anything, and Marj would describe what had happened.

The "What do you see?" "What do you notice?" practice taught a multitude of things. Observation—omniservation—wasn't solely a visual report: sight, sound, sense of movement, or impressions of changes in communication or thought or presence were all key components in answering these questions. The student having the turn might further report on elements such as thinking processes and emotional shifts. This questioning practice facilitated analysis, not only in the lesson you were watching, but also within your own process.

That each of us was asked to verbalize what we noticed, both in our own and others' turns, helped us take ownership of the learning. As simple as this interchange was, these questions proved a powerful learning tool for all involved.

In the Living Room Étude, Marj expected you to be an expert omniserver and fluent reporter of yourself as well as your students. Your ability to constructively answer "What do you notice about yourself?" and "What do you notice about your student(s)?" was an absolute requirement.

Impression Six: Constructive Thinking

Relentless constructive thinking.

Constructive derives from the word *construct*: putting things together to create something. This is how I understand *constructive* in relationship to F.M. Alexander's discoveries—as the diligent step-by-step process to achieve what I want.

As I undertook my studies, I had no idea that Marj was consistently modeling an approach to thinking that was indeed a "delicate revolution" in my psyche. In learning to teach, constructive thinking was the turning point for me in my encounter with the Living Room Étude. I left one of those Tuesday evening classes deeply frustrated, tears streaming, once again not getting anywhere near my student, once again "thinking about that for a while."

After an evening of renewed soul-self-searching, the answer emerged. I realized that every time Marj stopped me that evening and asked, "What do you notice about yourself?" "What do you notice about your student?" I had been thinking something nonconstructive—something hypercritical and unkind about myself. I was elated with this discovery, for now I knew what I had to do. "If I want to teach, I am going to need to learn to think constructively all the way across the room." Although it was still some months before I actually got to my student, I was never frustrated by this again—I knew my job. Marj trusted me; she had always held that this work was something that I could do, that I would succeed at, that learning was pleasurable, fun, and effective. Even in my deepest moments of frustration, I never thought I could fail.

Impression Seven: Rediscovery of The Use of the Self

During a month-long residency at a training school, the students expressed confusion about the moment-to-moment choices in teaching a lesson. They were ready to start teaching but had no idea how to begin. I was puzzled. I knew that I knew how to teach a lesson, and that effectively organizing the time was clear and easy for me. However, I found that I had never specifically articulated what I was doing. In retrospect, I recognize that Marj modeled a terrific teaching process. As someone teaching teachers, I desired to give words to that process.

I proposed that each day, I would analyze step by step what I thought I was doing while teaching the class. Preparing for Day Eight, I laughed as I recognized the sequence that had emerged. When I presented the full chart to the training group that evening, I asked, "Do you see what we have discovered?" What had been revealed was a mini outline of F.M. Alexander's seminal chapter "Evolution of a Technique" in his book *The Use of the Self.*

The steps I discovered on each day:

Day One Desire: "What do I want?"

Day Two Recognizing: The thing that has driven the lesson request.

Day Three Deciding: "Do I want to make a change?"

Day Four Gathering and selecting information.

Day Five Creating a plan.

Day Six Asking for that plan.

Day Seven Renewing freedom of choice (if necessary).

Day Eight Experimenting/taking the plan into action.

In these steps, I saw F.M. Alexander's story:

- F.M. Alexander wanted to speak Shakespeare. (Desire)

- He recognized that his voice was not working very well. (Recognizing)

- He wanted to figure out how to solve his issues. (Deciding)

- He observed himself speaking and not speaking, hypothesized what was happening and what might help, and tested his ideas over and over again. (Gathering and selecting information, Creating a plan, Experimenting/taking the plan into action)

- When necessary, he renewed his freedom to choose.

If you could have seen Marj's copy of *The Use of the Self*, you would realize how many times she turned and mulled over those pages. This is the one book she consistently asked us to read. I remember that the first time I read "Evolution of a Technique," the Victorian prose seemed obscure. After neglecting this chapter for a few years, when I opened the pages again, I was shocked to realize that I was reading along as if it was contemporary English. All that I had learned during my years with Marj had changed my relationship to the material.

My sequence of teaching matched F.M. Alexander's story in that first chapter. What I now refer to as the *Alexander Technique Progression* (AT Progression) turned out to be the dynamic scaffolding of my teaching.

Chapter 2

MY PERSPECTIVE ON THE ALEXANDER TECHNIQUE

My current "fancy" definition of the Alexander Technique:

Constructive conscious kindness to yourself
Cooperating with your design
Serving your desires and dreams.

My desire and intention is to teach people to use the Alexander Technique for themselves. This book's focus is on teaching the Alexander Technique rather than knowing or learning the Alexander Technique. Understanding how I approach this work, however, is necessary background for integrating the material I present on teaching.

A comprehensive discussion of my Alexander Technique perspective and process can be found in my book *Integrative Alexander Technique Practice for Performing Artists: Onstage Synergy* (Madden 2014).

What I Hope People Learn When I Teach the Alexander Technique

- In vertebrate coordination, the head–spine relationship in movement can either facilitate a cooperating coordination or cause interference in carrying out desired actions.

- We can consciously cooperate with the coordinating movement of the head in relationship to the spine to optimize our efficacy.

- The process to expedite a cooperating coordination, which I call the *AT Progression*, includes these steps:

— Wanting: You have a desire to do something, say something, think something.

— Recognizing: Something causes you to wonder about your coordination.

— Deciding: You decide to explore alternate choices.

— Gathering Information: You ask yourself questions about how you are doing what you are doing; you ask yourself questions about the circumstances in which you are doing it; you ask yourself questions about the activity itself; you may need to consult other resources, such as anatomy, specialized skill techniques, and so forth.

— Creating a Plan: Using this information, you make a new plan that first includes a specific instruction to your whole self in order to do what you are doing. The words I use to represent this process throughout this text are "Ask yourself to COORDINATE so that your head can move so that all of you can follow so that you can do what you are doing."

— Asking: You volitionally ask yourself to carry out the new plan.

— Acting/Experimenting: You carry out the new plan.

• A constructive plan for the Alexander process includes the wish for what I call the coordinating organization ("I ask myself to COORDINATE so that my head can move so that all of me can follow...") seamlessly connected to the wish for whatever activity you are doing ("...so that I can do what I am doing"). If the coordination organizing wish is not directly connected to doing something, the result is usually an overall discoordination.

• Learning to integrate the Alexander Technique in your life involves developing many new studied rehearsed plans.

• The work directly relates to your whole life. For performers, I developed an overall template, acknowledging that using the Alexander Technique has a whole-self-in-a-whole-world intent:

I use the Alexander Technique
to use the techniques of my art form
along with my performance skills
to invite this audience on this journey
...for a specific reason
...for my artistic purpose
...to serve my life and the world.

This template can be modified to suit any of life's tasks. For instance:

I use the Alexander Technique
to use what I have learned about arm movement
to pick up this glass of water
to hydrate myself
so that I have the requisite energy
to serve my life and the world.

For More Detail

I also recommend the aforementioned "Evolution of a Technique" chapter in F.M. Alexander's book *The Use of the Self* (1984[1932]). Many books with introductory material are available, and my book and F.M. Alexander's chapter most clearly match my approach to the work. Please note that F.M. Alexander's chapter, although excellent, is rife with "goods," "bads," "rights," and "wrongs." I have adapted for myself a version that uses as many of the original words as possible while eliminating those judgmental, "no"-oriented word choices.

All Teaching Is Group Teaching

I don't approach lessons with the smallest possible group (two: myself and the student) much differently than larger group lessons. The processes are much the same. While I offer ideas pertinent to each of these ways of teaching, please note that I regard the underlying intent and many of the processes as exactly the same.

Cathy Glossary

My experiments with words have their origin in my study with Marj. She was always looking for better ways to teach the work, including examining the words she used. I first played with word choice while teaching an adult acting class at the Community Theatre in Lincoln. I was not yet able to teach the Alexander Technique, but I was noticing how my students were moving and how they reacted to different words. I actively experimented with words that would bring forth the optimal response. For quick reference, following are key terms that I have integrated into my personal teaching vocabulary (some of which have already appeared in this book).

AT Progression

Throughout the book, I use this to refer to the steps referred to earlier, distilling the narrative F.M. Alexander described in *The Use of the Self*: Wanting, Recognizing, Deciding, Gathering Information, Creating a Plan, then carrying out the plan, inviting yourself to action knowing that you have freedom to choose.

Back-Pocket Plan

When I encounter a recurring situation or an activity in which I perceive, "Every time this happens, I tighten between head and spine," I research a new way to respond to the event. I devise an Alexander Technique-facilitated new plan to have in place, enabling me to respond in coordination rather than by tightening as soon I realize that the situation is about to recur.

Biopsychosocial

A relative newcomer to my vocabulary is this alternate to the *psychophysical unity* often seen in Alexander Technique discussions; *biopsychosocial* seems more inclusive to me. As its components suggest, the term encompasses the interaction of biological, psychological, and social elements in our coordination.

Constructive

In the last chapter, I connected this term to the verb *construct*. It is the quality of the "yes" plan, the pursuit of what you want, building step by step to a goal.

Coordination

The quality of our coordination is determined by many factors, and the Alexander Technique seeks to optimize those factors in facilitating our search for excellence. The sense in which I mean to COORDINATE is to call a harmonious organization of the whole self to the parts and the parts to the whole self. *Coordination* further describes how all aspects of who we are contribute to our accomplishing whatever we are doing. At the Performance School, a center for the study of the Alexander Technique that I co-founded in Seattle, our definition was emblazoned on one of our brochures: "Coordination is the ability to conceive of an idea and carry that idea out as conceived."

Design

Design is my way of referring to how all our systems are organized to function when working optimally. It encompasses all the elements of our biopsychosocial selves—structural, emotional, intellectual, relational, and so on.

Hinankle

In discussing whole-leg movement, I often said, "hip, knee, ankle, and a bunch of stuff in your feet." One of my students was tired of repeatedly hearing all these words and coined "hinankle." I include it here as an example of a student-contributed word.

Invented Verb

I often have my students create a made-up verb that means "Invite myself to cooperate with my design." Some of the many we have used: *Lumaria, Allaly, Upsolé, Mytilus, Anemonize, Rakusa, Imini, Buzzaloo, Echrisal, Pysaster, P'ching,* and *Zing-ha*. In this book, I use COORDINATE in small capitals to indicate this volitional invitational verb.

Kindness

Using *kindness* to describe teaching became part of my vocabulary after I studied with the Cree Elder Eddie Belrose. When I learned that honesty and kindness—first to yourself, then to others—are the rules of the Cree Nation, I realized that these are integral watchwords of my teaching.

I was recently introduced to Daniel Siegel's work, and his definition of kindness also speaks to me: "The visible, natural outcome of integration. Positive regard for others, compassionate intention, and acts of extending oneself in service of others are all different manifestations of the differentiation and linkage of selves within a larger 'We' at the heart of being kind. Involves honoring and supporting the vulnerability of others and the self" (2012, pp.41–44).

Minking and Thoving

Introduced earlier, this is another phrase with a teaching-need origin: A student's conception of self was so disjointed that we couldn't even say *think* or *move* without causing discoordination. Hence, we scrambled the words into *minking* and *thoving*.

Omniservation

Observation is a key component of any teaching process. But all that I experience in my student is not only about vision, but rather receiving through all my senses. The word *observation* tends to cause people to think solely visually. So, I coined *omniservation* to emphasize that many senses are involved.

Quick Walks

These originated in the Nebraska workshops with Marj. They are simply walking turns during which the teacher uses their hands in teaching for just a moment as students file past—everyone experimenting with walking.

Studied Rehearsed Plan

Studied rehearsed plans are developed skills that serve a desired action. For the Alexander Technique, the plan generally takes the form: "Ask myself to COORDINATE so that my head can move so that all of me can follow so that I can do what I am doing." In practice, the "do what I am doing" phrase is given as much detail as needed or appropriate to the task at hand.

Turn

While not unique to me, this term appears often enough in the book that it deserves mention. A "turn" is the central unit in how I teach the Alexander Technique: A student asks a question, a process is engaged to answer the question, and a constructive plan emerges. In group classes, people often talk about taking turns.

Part Two

ESSENTIAL SKILLS FOR TEACHING THE ALEXANDER TECHNIQUE

Chapter 3

THE FLOW OF TEACHING

What Is Teaching?

For as long as I have defined it, *teaching* has meant "creating the conditions in which my students can learn what they want to learn." When searching for the potential source of this definition, I found it attributed (with no original sourcing) to Albert Einstein: "'I never *teach* my pupils. I only attempt to provide the conditions in which they can learn'" (King 1964, p.126). Perhaps I read those words somewhere, and recognizing both my values and the way in which teachers I respected taught, I adopted and adapted it.

"Creating the conditions in which someone can learn" encompasses many things I do—from providing information, to choreographing a dance so someone can practice receiving choreography, to giving a lecture on the physiology of emotions, to calling on my training as a childbirth educator. Everything I accumulate in knowledge and experience contributes to the moment of teaching the Alexander Technique. Lessons vary from teacher to teacher, modulated by our unique knowledge and experience. How the students' needs dance with our distinctive selves enriches the learning environment.

My addition to Einstein's attributed quote is "what they want to learn," which harks back to the "I want to teach!" impression from the Living Room Étude. Every lesson with Marj exercised student desire. As you'll hear repeatedly, student desire also leads my teaching.

Teaching is creating the conditions in which my students can learn what they want to learn.

What Is Teaching the Alexander Technique?

Teaching the Alexander Technique is about using your skills and knowledge to provide the information people need to consciously use the Alexander Technique to do what they are doing, learning how to develop new plans for themselves as new situations arise. From the beginning, I enable people to experiment on their own. As their facility develops, my job is to create the conditions in which they can achieve the next level of expertise.

When I teach acting, my definition of teaching remains: "Creating the conditions in which my student(s) can learn what they want to learn." What is required of me changes. Although I might demonstrate something about acting when I teach it, I am generally not acting while teaching acting. (It is amusing to think of some of the characters I have played as acting teachers, but I don't think they'd be so good at it.) However, while I could offer information about the Alexander Technique without actively using it, teaching the Alexander Technique effectively absolutely requires that I use it while teaching it.

Our "Self" in Teaching

In an interview with Marj, Joan Schirle (1987, p.6) asked, "Is that what you're trying to get teachers to do—exactly what they are telling their students to do?" Marj answered, "The teachers really must be able to do it in order to teach it to the students…this is what I've found out." The intent of the Living Room Étude is to teach this skill.

Using the Alexander Technique facilitates quality in our coordination, bringing quality to whatever we choose to do in teaching. We are "walking our talk." Countless admonitions about teaching emphasize that the teacher's self is the real teacher. Of the many I could cite, I quote Palmer:

> teaching holds a mirror to the soul. If I am willing to look in that mirror and not run from what I see, I have a chance to gain

TEACHING STORY

In the process of teaching us to teach, Cathy often stressed the notion that we needed to actually want to teach—and raise our hands and say it—in order to have a lesson from her that involved teaching.

I absolutely recognize the wisdom of this on many levels, but first and foremost, Cathy wanted us to use the Alexander Technique in an activity to learn this new skill. Desire is the first piece of this.

By the time I raised my hand and said clearly, "I want to teach," I had built up so much energy behind that wish that when I got the go-ahead from Cathy, I shot across the room toward my student, Carol Levin, who—sensibly—backed herself up against the wall. Takeaway: What do you notice about yourself?

self-knowledge—and knowing myself is as crucial to good teaching as knowing my students and my subject... When I do not know myself, I cannot know my subject—not at the deepest levels of embodied, personal meaning. I will know it only abstractly, from a distance, a congeries of concepts as far removed from the world as I am from personal truth... Good teaching requires self-knowledge: it is a hidden secret in plain sight. (Palmer 1998, pp.2–3)

The burgeoning field of neuroscience has been exciting for me as an educator because research studies are starting to provide the science supporting long-used teaching techniques. Caution is a watchword as I read new studies, having been schooled by scientists that new work is constantly evolving; yet some of the emerging work illuminates common practices. The work with mirror neurons, for instance, supports our need to use the Alexander Technique in order to teach the Alexander Technique. Sandra and Matthew Blakeslee, reporting on the current research about body maps, define mirror neurons as "a special set of cells within certain high-level body maps that represent actions performed both by oneself and by others; hence, they are key to many higher mental functions, including imitation, empathy, and the ability to read one another's intentions" (Blakeslee and Blakeslee 2007, p.213).

It is these imitative functions that we serve when using what we know in order to teach. While mirror neurons are only one aspect of imitation, and research is ongoing on how imitation happens at different ages and stages, everyone knows that imitation has an educational function. Whether learning how to button our clothes, throw a ball, or dance a tango, we have all experienced learning something by imitating someone else doing it. And this is true as well of how people learn the Alexander Technique. As teachers, we are the model of the change process.

The first time I demonstrated using the Alexander Technique in front of a class, consciously using imitation as a teaching tool, relentless constructive thinking replaced my fear of demonstrating. Relatively rapidly, probably due to all the constructive planning I needed to do to accomplish it, demonstrating became normal. This is important because some students learn most easily via demonstration. A student in a weekly class reported that she was more comfortable sleeping (and, in fact, so was her whole household) after the lesson in sleeping she'd had the week before. I recalled that she had watched rather than participated in that section of the class. She explained, "Oh yes, I learn much better by watching rather than taking a turn myself." Today, when so many people are primed to learn visually because of the prevalence of computers, phones, tablets, and other electronic devices, the ability to model using the Alexander Technique is more important than ever.

Knowing that people may model me has guided me in a variety of ways. For example, I was teaching in Japan after injuring my left knee. When going to sit on the floor, I needed to find a way to get down there without bending the knee. My plan was working well, but I noticed a few people going to the floor using my temporarily necessary way. I reminded everyone that, while getting to the floor without bending your knee is always an option if desired, it is not required for the activity.

A humorous example was with a student who was learning to teach the Alexander Technique. Every time he taught someone, he would go into a fairly deep knee bend. I pointed out that, while he was doing this with good coordination, it wasn't necessary and looked a bit odd. One day, when teaching a student who was taller than him, he was still bending his knees deeply even though this made it more difficult to use his hands to reach his student. When I pointed this out, he started laughing—suddenly, he realized he was imitating me to the point of trying to match my height.

Stages of Teaching the Alexander Technique

In one workshop for teachers and people learning to teach, my participants were already experts. However, they kept evaluating themselves as less capable than they were. As I puzzled over this, a theory of three general stages in learning the Alexander Technique emerged.

Stage One: What Is the Alexander Technique?

During this time, learning involves acquiring a necessary systemic accumulation of information, theory, principles, and beginning practice in using the work. During this stage, the teacher, while still needing to elicit the desire of the student, tends to be in the lead. (Beginner)

Stage Two: Studied Rehearsed Plan Practice/Accumulation

By using Stage One material in a variety of circumstances, learners develop a vocabulary of studied rehearsed plans. The teacher's task moves from creating studied rehearsed plans with the student to teaching the student how to create them for themselves. I think of this as "practicing to confidence." (Intermediate)

Stage Three: Skill Building/Integrative Practice

Sustaining the use of the Alexander Technique over more and more time in increasingly complex ways as well as becoming fluent in combining studied rehearsed plans in series is the task of Stage Three. In this stage, the job of the teacher is to provide feedback, primarily teaching the student how to do the detective and coordination work on their own, while still supplying necessary feedback and information. (Expert)

For the aforementioned workshop, I drew a chart on the board. After every lesson, we marked which stage the lesson matched (some lessons spanned two stages). If 16 lessons had taken place, the chart might look like Table 3.1.

Table 3.1 Stages of Learning the Alexander Technique

Stage One	Stage Two	Stage Three
✓✓✓✓	✓✓✓✓✓✓✓✓	✓✓✓✓

Filling in the chart revealed for these advanced students that they weren't giving themselves credit for what they already knew. They were judging their Stage Three questions as if they were Stage One questions, leading to disparaging assessments of their own skills. Once the class evaluated themselves in a way appropriate to their true stage of learning, they were much more constructive in utilizing new information.

A current influence in my teaching is Ericsson's research on expert performance. In his book, co-written with Robert Pool, *Peak: Secrets from the New Science of Expertise* (2016), he identifies the characteristics of what he calls deliberate practice, which parallel elements of my three stages of learning the Alexander Technique. Noting that deliberate practice relies on an expert teacher/coach as a guide, here is how his ideas correspond to the three stages:

Stage One: "Deliberate practice develops skills that other people have already figured out how to do and for which effective training techniques have already been developed" (Ericsson and Pool 2016, p.99).

Stage Two: "Deliberate practice involves well-defined, specific goals and often involves improving some aspect of the target performance... Once an overall goal has been set, a teacher or coach will develop a plan for making a series of small changes that will add up to the desired larger change" (Ericsson and Pool 2016, p.99).

Stage Three: "Deliberate practice involves feedback and modifications of efforts in response to that feedback. Early in the training process much of the feedback will come from the teacher or coach... With time and experience students must learn to monitor themselves, spot mistakes, and adjust accordingly" (Ericsson and Pool 2016, p.99).

(*Note*: A more detailed discussion of Ericsson's deliberate practice in relationship to the Alexander Technique is the subject of Chapter 17.)

Teaching Template

Some years ago, a group of people were having difficulty figuring out what their job was in becoming a teacher. A few of them were asking to teach but not taking charge of integrating their Stage Two learning into a teaching plan. None of my suggestions seemed to be getting through. One night, seeking a new idea, I used many sticky notes to chart my sequential plan for teaching. When the class arrived the next day, the board was filled with sticky notes, detailing the steps in my process. Figure 3.1 is based on my sticky-note creation.

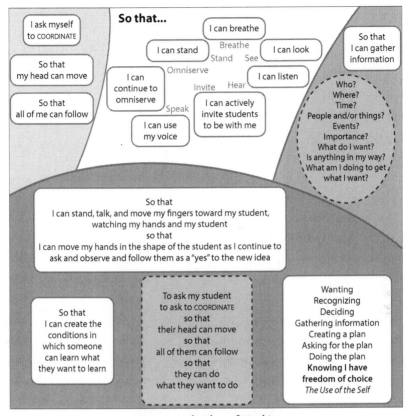

Figure 3.1 The Flow of Teaching

In rereading Marj's Preface to the Centerline Press edition of *The Use of the Self*, I recognized what my chart illustrates:

> The most remarkable aspect of F.M. experiments proved that the only true guidance needed was his sequence of directional thinking which must carry through no matter what movement is to be accomplished. Professor John Dewey termed this aspect "thinking in activity."
>
> Both F.M. Alexander and (his brother and teaching partner) A.R. Alexander stressed the sequence of directional thinking in their teaching. At times, they seemed almost too persistent on this point, but really they were not. This *new* way of thinking and this *new* approach to learning was so unfamiliar it required constant reinforcement. (Alexander 1984[1932])

Chapter 4

THE LEARNING PLAYGROUND

For education, we need a teacher, a student, and a space for the interaction to happen—what I think of as a learning playground. Acknowledging that the primary dynamic in an Alexander Technique learning event is the relationship between teacher and student (detailed in subsequent chapters), I first set the scene by offering some thoughts on the physical environment of teaching. A class, a lesson, a workshop—all are first defined by having a time and place to meet.

The Classroom as a Place to Play

Diane Ackerman, whose book *Deep Play* significantly helped me understand how I used play in teaching, notes: "Play always has a sacred place—some version of a playground—in which it happens. The hallowed ground is usually outlined so that it's clearly set off from the rest of reality. This place may be a classroom…" (1999, p.6).

Joyful experimentation is facilitated when it is understood that a key characteristic of the adult classroom is its separation from "real life."

My Teaching Studio

As I sit in the open space in the middle of my home studio, I see an upright piano loaned to the studio by a friend, my father's leather sofa and chair, a high stool, and a selection of other wooden chairs. A lamp that was a gift from my mother sits on a desk that was my grandmother's vanity. A bookshelf holds my books for sale as well as a variety of toys. A bunch of bones spill over the edge of a basket onto the floor. Two coffee tables from my childhood home serve as bookshelves for a collection of anatomy books and some poetry chapbooks (written by my students Carol Levin and Deborah Green). The John Hopkins articulated skeleton and three beautiful, meticulously crafted pipe cleaner skeletons fashioned by my student, Ken Anno, also sit on the tables. A filing cabinet holds more toys; several hula hoops are propped up against it. Many pipe cleaner creations adorn the room, including a rainbow orca and one of my cat driving a vintage car with wheels that move. Another student, Shoko Zama, has contributed three paintings: a beautiful abstract angel-looking figure that looks over the room from the piano; a large, colorful abstract piece; and, in the corner, an ink drawing depicting a string quartet whose movement she had admired. Also on the walls are two photos of me, one teaching on a hill in Rheinfelden, Switzerland, and the other giving a speech at the Freiburg Congress, and a larger photo of Marj. Other prints illustrate Oregon coast waves and a whimsical Galway florist. The light switch plate is painted with small purple flowers, with two wall stickers of tiny people "holding" the plate up. Free weights, kettle bells, a golf club, a step unit, a ukulele, and bits of toys peep out from the corner of the room. You can see shelves of books in the hallway just beyond the studio. A large window looks out into a garden and across a small ravine filled with evergreen trees.

TEACHING STORY

In class, my activity was to prepare for the public reading of my own poetry I was scheduled to give. The particular poem I was concerned about had verses of text, alternating with snippets of songs that I planned to sing. I am not a singer.

I faced the class, read the text, and sang the songs, then sighed in order to take a full breath and relieve all the clutching I was doing. Cathy suggested I play around, talk the songs, and sing the text verses. What?! And then I did. All of a sudden, I was having sooooo much fun that I was dancing along with myself. And my audience was totally with me. Grinning.

Now, when I prepare for readings, I sing my poems a few times to warm up and it feels like everything pops open. I'm still having fun.

My space vibrantly expresses that I invite experimentation and play in as many varieties of activity as possible. (Because the studio is part of my home, I have more props and resources for activities than are visible in the room.) Many objects in the room are intentionally humorous. It isn't as large or high a space as I'd really prefer, but a home studio helps keep the cost of classes and lessons reasonable and obviously is convenient. (I can rent space elsewhere if I need a different environment.) Because my studio is relatively small, I have experimented with ways to arrange the room to encourage movement. The open area in the middle visually invites activity. Formerly, students could see a fireplace on the back wall. For some reason, no one would sit on that side of the room, even without a fire, so I effectively lost half of what space I had. The piano now covers the fireplace, and I can use the whole room. Many lessons take place facing the large window, which brings the outside into the space, making it feel larger.

I was additionally inspired by the aesthetics of the Seattle Waldorf School (Steiner School), which features lots of rounded shapes. When you are in any Steiner-inspired building, you see immediately that most of the corners are rounded. He wanted architecture to reflect nature, which has no straight edges. The teachers even round the corners of all the paper the children use. I look for ways to minimize or slightly disguise the corners of square rooms in such a way that they can flow. One of my paintings, for instance, is hung at an angle across the corner. A lamp with a rounded shape is in another corner. Presenting curves rather than straight lines changes the moving atmosphere of the room. I endeavor to create a learning environment that flows and is rich with stimuli and possibility.

Malcolm Knowles, an American educator recognized as the leader in defining principles of adult learning (andragogy), discusses "establishing a climate conducive to learning," noting that beyond the basic human comfort needs, ecological psychologists offer "valuable information about the effects of the physical properties of environment on learning" (Knowles, Holton, and Swanson 2005, p.118). This includes color, with brighter colors not surprisingly offering a more cheerful atmosphere. He tested this with a weekly group meeting that was not "clicking in the way most classes do" (Knowles *et al.* 2005, p.118). As an experiment, some of the members of the group spent a small amount of money on materials to "make collages for the walls, mobiles for the ceiling and simulated flagstones for the floor. What a happier mood characterized the next meeting!" (Knowles *et al.* 2005, p.119).

I am a theatre director. Part of the job description is to create a ground plan for the actors to play in that encourages movement and dynamic stage pictures, inviting an audience into the story. I am adept at looking at a space and seeing how it encourages communication. What I refer to as a space that moves, ecological psychologists describe as "concern for environmental facilitation of interaction among the learners" (Knowles *et al.* 2005, p.119).

My studio—with its wide variety of tools and toys—exemplifies what Knowles *et al.* describe in this passage: "another aspect of the environment that all theorists agree is crucial to effective learning is the richness and accessibility of resources—both material and human... The important thing is not just that these resources are available but that learners can use them pro-actively" (2005, p.119). I want students to use the Alexander Technique immediately in the tasks of their daily life; thus, I do my best to set up an environment to constantly encourage integrative activities.

When the Classroom Isn't Solely Yours

I describe my studio in such detail because it is the environment over which I have the most control. While I have ideas to improve it, and recognize that it is a little casual for some of my students who might prefer a more "ordered" milieu, it serves me well. My taller students adapt to the low ceiling, and I can generally make the space work for anyone through how I interact with them in it.

Taking charge of your space, adapting as necessary, is often the first thing you do when teaching—before the students arrive. As you arrive in your teaching space, evaluate its movement potential by asking, "Do I sense movement in this space?" or "Do I want to move in this space?" If you don't feel encouraged to move and explore, ask yourself, "What elements can I change?" Most of the time, simple solutions can positively alter the environment.

When creating a space that moves well for learning, I look for light—opening windows and turning on lights as needed. I create curves in the room when possible, particularly in the corners. Noting that symmetry tends to make a room more static, I strategically create some unevenness. I love teaching in a space that has windows to nature, which then becomes part of the indoor environment. In a shared setting, I take my own anatomy reference books and teaching props such as juggling balls and writing supplies with me to class, and have been known to purchase colorful toys during a break if the room needs a little "pep."

During my early teaching days in Nebraska, when we assisted Marj at large workshops, the assistants would teach in "breakout rooms," which tended to be oddly shaped rooms in the University of Nebraska dormitories, with platforms instead of chairs. My adaptability to environment in teaching may have its origins in those teaching sessions. Following are a few anecdotes about adjusting a teaching space as needed to facilitate learning.

One particularly challenging room was a completely square space with a bank of lights housed in a completely square shape on the ceiling. The circle of chairs for my participants was enclosed by a square above them and a square around them. During the first session, everyone was struggling with accepting new ideas, and I could hardly get anyone to take a turn or even ask a question. At the tea break, I thought about it, then rearranged the chairs into an egg shape, extending beyond the ceiling-defined square. I also left the door open. In this modified configuration, the class moved more smoothly. Then someone closed the door—and we got stuck again. I had to explain that keeping the door open, while not necessarily the custom of that group, was helping the learning process.

A space I regularly teach in greets you with a large skeleton as you enter. Although I use anatomy in my teaching, I prefer that a skeleton not be the first thing someone sees when arriving for my class. So, I move the skeleton to another room, where it is accessible but not immediately visible.

At an acting studio in Seattle, with no preplanning, all of the students arrived with combs, hair dryers, razors, soap, and make-up. We relocated our learning space by moving down the hall, putting a sign on the door indicating our willingness to leave, and holding class in the women's bathroom.

If something is "off" in the environment and you can't fix it, the easiest way to make it less of an obstacle to learning is simply to acknowledge it. I once taught a workshop that was ridiculously crowded—the participants literally filled at least 90 percent of the floor space. I just acknowledged these circumstances, and each time we had to carve out a bit more room for someone's turn, we varied which side of the room got to be "squished." Playing with the obstacle made it serve rather than hinder the teaching.

Respond to your environment—use what works, change what doesn't if you can.

Chapter 5

ALEXANDER TECHNIQUE PROGRESSION

I began this story in Chapter 1 when discussing the Living Room Étude. Teaching the Alexander Technique is something I just seemed to know how to do. I hadn't analyzed my teaching process until a group of students learning to teach asked, "How do you know what to do and when to do it in a lesson?" I remember asking something to the effect of, "You don't know what to do?" Silence. "I seem to know what to do as it happens—it just makes sense to me."

I realized that my working understanding of the Alexander Technique teaching process developed from watching Marj teach. While this was sufficient for my personal teaching practice, in order to teach people to teach, I needed to be able to articulate what I was doing. My offer to the class was to research over the next week what I thought I was doing, reporting what I found out. This week of investigation (described in the first chapter) led to what I sometimes call the world's shortest version of *The Use of the Self.*

My wording of the sequence has varied slightly over time and by situation. Generally, I express the steps in the form of "-ing," which can be a gerund (noun that names the step) or a present participle (verb form used to express continuous actions over time). The "-ing" accomplishes both naming the step and signifying a process that flows over time.

Here again is the list of steps I distilled from my teaching findings, this time explained in relationship to F.M. Alexander's chapter "Evolution of a Technique."

The AT Progression

Wanting: Alexander wanted to speak Shakespeare.

Recognizing: He recognized that he was having trouble with his voice.

Deciding: He decided to investigate what was happening and search for solutions.

Gathering Information: He gathered information to figure out what to do.

Creating a Plan: He used the information to create a plan for speaking.

Asking: He asked himself to carry out the plan.

Acting/Experimenting: He spoke.

This process all takes place within the context of freedom of choice. If necessary, a Deciding Again step can be added at any time.

What I sometimes call "The Desire Trio"—Wanting, Recognizing, Deciding—derive from F.M. Alexander's story, though they are perhaps the most forgotten of the steps in the AT Progression. Without this trio, however, nothing else happens. Without desire, recognition, and decision, no one would ever show up to class. If F.M. Alexander had not had a burning desire to speak Shakespeare, the Alexander Technique would not have been created.

The process of a lesson is not as linear as the AT Progression list looks; lessons generally flow through all of these steps multiple times. A typical flow in a lesson might be...

- Wanting
  - Recognizing
    - Deciding
      - Gathering information
        - Creating a plan
          - Being inspired by the plan to gather more information

- Creating a new plan that again creates a need for gathering information
  - Updating the plan according to all of this information
    - Carrying out the plan
      - This fuels a desire to gather more information
        - Perhaps needing to decide again
          - Thus creating a new plan
            - Acting/doing this plan
              - And so on...

Teaching Considerations for Each Step

Wanting

Many teachers have asked me, "What if my students say they don't want anything?" Once people have organized their lives to come to your studio at a specific time and date, it is safe to assume they want something. Articulating desire is one of the first things I teach. Very rarely does someone arrive at a class, workshop, or lesson who hasn't thought about why they are coming—because they have learned that I will ask.

Here are some of the many ways to wake up desire if it happens to be sleeping:

- "What brought you here today?"
- "Is there anything you are interested in looking at?"
- "What is the next step on your journey?"
- "Do you want to do this or this?" (Offering choices—they are still the ones who decide.)
- "Do you want to _____?" (Offering a single choice, still asking them to decide.)
- "I've been thinking about arm movement." (Or something else.) "Would anyone like to experiment with how you move your arm above your head?"

- You could offer a game. (In "Games Digest," I note several games that work well at the beginning of a class.)

- You could read a text about the Alexander Technique or related to the Alexander Technique, then ask if anyone has a response to the text.

When I held my weekly class at 5:30 p.m., many people were arriving from their workday. I found that asking them if they wanted quick walks (and waiting for "yes") helped everyone switch from work to play. By 5:37, an explosion of wants would arrive.

You are in search of the "yes." Without the "yes," offering information risks eliciting "I should" or "I have to" or "There is something wrong with me" relationships to learning.

Recognizing

For me, this step simply consists of whatever might have caused someone to think to use the Alexander Technique. It might be something you notice about yourself and/or something related to an activity you do. It might be something you've heard from someone else and decided to investigate. I emphasize that *recognizing* doesn't mean that something is going wrong. In my case, most of the time, what I recognize is that I am about to do something, and I've experienced that the Alexander Technique consistently helps me do what I want to do with enhanced quality. Consequently, I emphasize to my students that the Alexander Technique ultimately is about facilitating excellence—rather than fixing problems.

Deciding

Usually, the fact that someone has volunteered for a turn means that they have decided to explore the activity of their wanting/recognizing. I remain attentive to this throughout a lesson, particularly if it starts flowing in a different direction from the desire they expressed. I may ask again, "Is this what you want to explore?" For instance, sometimes a lesson starts to be about walking, but with analysis, the reason the legs are moving the way they are is coming from how the person is thinking about their arms. I will explain what I am thinking and either look for nonverbal assent or directly ask for it. Another example is if a lesson suddenly becomes more emotionally laden than anticipated—someone has asked to look at breathing and the exploration is successful in improving coordination but has also caused crying. I will respond to the emotions as might be appropriate, and also ask permission to continue.

Gathering Information

The "Omniservation," "Analysis of Activity," and "The Art of the Question" chapters present the primary skills needed for this step in the process. As we teach the Alexander Technique to help students explore the activity of their choice, we may also need to seek information from auxiliary fields. "I can do a little research on that" is an important offer in teaching.

The room I most loved in Marj's house was her study. I fondly recall a fireplace in the corner surrounded by tiles. Enclosed bookshelves. Dolls. The telephone that she most often used. And a revolving wagon wheel, glass-covered coffee table heaped with magazines. Some of these covered topics we knew Marj was interested in—horses, ranching, dolls. Every year, however, we noticed new magazines on new topics—some surprising. This was perhaps the first time I consciously recognized someone choosing to challenge herself with new ideas. Marj was an exemplar for us, inspiring us always to keep curious.

My research has led me into areas I never knew I'd care about. For example, I originally sought a personal trainer because so many of my students were doing weight training and I felt I didn't know enough about it. I discovered that it was fun and I liked it, so I have continued to this day. Curiosity is a superb aid in teaching the Alexander Technique.

Creating a Plan

I usually phrase the essential Alexander Technique plan:

> I ask myself to COORDINATE
> so that
> my head can move
> so that

all of me can follow
so that
I can do what I am doing.

The two continuous components are the message to the underlying coordination and the message(s) about the activity—what you are doing. This can be anything from sitting and breathing to climbing a mountain. The phrase "so that" is the causal conjunctive phrase that creates one seamless thought, one ask rather than two.

My use of the phrase "so that I can" probably derives from a book I read over and over again as a child—Watty Piper's 1930 story, *The Little Engine that Could.* The story tells of some railcars who need an engine to pull them over the mountain. Several engines, for differing reasons, choose not to help. Just as they are about to give up, the little blue engine, who happens to be a "she," arrives and, even though she isn't sure she can do it, agrees to help. She sounds her efforts in the repeated, rhythmic "I think I can..." Ultimately, she succeeds in getting over the mountain (Piper 2002[1930]).

For me, "I can" connotes an active, constructive process toward a goal that I expect to be successful. It acknowledges the ability or potential to do something while also connoting the free choice to continue to do it or choose another goal. When I am teaching, I need to make sure *can* is a constructive word for my students. For some people, *can* means something in the future rather than active right now. Some people think of "I can" as conjectural rather than an active request, so I am attentive to anything that looks passive. The "so that I can" is my way of teaching what Professor John Dewey called "thinking in activity."

I teach this process from the first class and find that when students are entrusted with it from the first day, their ability to think in activity, to think while they act, is immediate. It is true that more information and experience builds their ability to use the Alexander Technique in a wide range of activities, yet it is immediately usable—from the first lesson.

Asking

I ask myself to use the plan I have created. *Ask* means thinking about the plan willfully—with an intention of something happening. Asking invites response, invites movement. *And it is the one step we cannot do for our students.* They are the only ones who can mink and thove their plan. As teachers, we may need to coach them and teach them how to ask constructively. Ultimately, this step is all theirs.

Acting/Experimenting

Active asking moves the plan into action. We do what we intended in order to test out the plan. This may lead to completion of the exploration due to success. Or it may lead to further exploration because something in the plan needs further investigation. In the latter case, we may decide to gather more information in order to create another version of the plan. We may do this for as long as we like.

> *This full sequence takes place within the context of freedom of choice.*

Deciding Again

Unless informed otherwise, I assume that the student is functioning from freedom of choice. If they are not, then we need Deciding Again, the step F.M. Alexander describes as choosing to do what he intended to do, to do something else, or to do nothing. I consider this an optional step because, most of the time, my students don't need it—they are doing what they want to do. When they do need it, I offer the options slightly differently than Alexander. I describe the choices as doing what you intended to do, doing any of the many other things you could do (and choosing one to consider), or continuing to do what you are doing. Humans can never actually do nothing—we are at the very least breathing. If you insist on the impossible plan of doing nothing, you will tighten between head and spine.

Teaching Students to Do These Steps Themselves

In what I identified earlier as Stage One (What is the Alexander Technique?), I am leading the sequence for most new students. It is in Stage Two (Studied Rehearsed Plan Practice/Accumulation) that my task balances more to teaching them to do the detective work and make the plans themselves.

From the first lesson, I verbally highlight these steps. People experience themselves and others using the sequence multiple times. As they become ready, I invite more and more active participation in the gathering information and plan creation phase of their lesson. "What information do you have?" "What information do you think you need?" "How would you use the information to get what you want?" "Is your plan constructive? Possible? Within your control?" and so on.

Supplemental written material such as handouts and books are often helpful here as well.

Learning Structure Games

Following are some games that illustrate the process and teach people to use the sequence themselves. Once people have done these, they tend to omniserve the AT Progression more in their own and others' lessons.

The Aerobic Version

I make signs with the names of each of the steps, then put them in different places around the room. While the class is watching the turn, they walk or run to the sign indicating whatever part of the process they think is occurring in the lesson. As lessons often progress rapidly, the activity quickly becomes aerobic.

TEACHING STORY

As part of my training for ATI Teacher Certification from 1999 to 2002, I arranged for Cathy to give a series of workshops for performers at Willamette University in Oregon, where I taught music. In the very first workshop, Cathy taught us to formulate and articulate a "plan of action" that should precede all activities. The plan was based on the sequential nature of Alexander's process. Students were encouraged to conceive plans that clarified their intentions leading up to actually beginning the activity. Plans could be more or less inclusive depending on where each student was in their learning process. The last part of the plan always pertained to the performer's ultimate goal: "*so that* I may express the music." Plans were personal and specific to the needs and issues of individual students.

In nearly 20 years of teaching a college course on the Alexander Technique to musicians and actors, having students formulate and articulate their plans in advance of performing has become a foundational element in my teaching. The process of formulating a plan, carrying it out, assessing its success, and then reformulating or adjusting the plan taught students the means for progressing to a higher standard all on their own.

The More Sedate Version

I make the same signs as in the aerobic version. This time, however, small groups of people are each given a sign, and their task is to watch the lesson from the perspective of that step in the process. After the lesson, the groups talk: Did they see the step? At what point? How many times did it repeat?

The Handout Version

I give each student several copies of the handout shown in Table 5.1, asking them to fill it in describing one of their own lessons as well as several other lessons they omniserved. Students can also use this sheet for between-session experiments.

Table 5.1 AT Progression Worksheet

Steps	Frequency	Description
Wanting		
Recognizing		
Deciding		
Gathering Information		
Creating a New Plan		
Asking/Experimenting		
Deciding Again (if applicable)		
Experimenting		

Chapter 6

WHOLE-SELF INVITATION

The Alexander Technique examines not what you do per se, but *how* you do what you do. When we consider any of the activities involved in teaching, we are searching for plans for those activities designed constructively, enabling us to sustain our overall coordination. Nonconstructive or impossible plans will cause us to discoordinate, even if we precede them with using the Alexander Technique. Asking to coordinate so that we can follow a constructive plan sustains our coordination. Using the Alexander Technique so that we can follow a nonconstructive plan causes us to tighten between head and spine; we may have an overall better quality of coordination than before, but we are still compromised. Our coordination serves as a barometer of constructive versus nonconstructive choice. Hence, using the Alexander Technique to select and use constructive, effective communication tools is a potent tool for communication in teaching—and in life.

Communication as Invitation

Acting was my first playground for Alexander Technique exploration— first for myself, then as an acting teacher and director in service of others, then as an Alexander Technique teacher serving theatre artists. While living in Lincoln, I founded and ran an acting company, Washington Street Players Place. Many of our shows were original pieces that we developed together or new works from our playwright Peg Sheldrick. In addition to performing, we held weekly company meetings to hone our skills. My primary objective in these classes was to experiment with deeply integrating the Alexander Technique and acting. Because acting imitates life, this also turned out to be a great playground for integrating the Alexander Technique with all kinds of communication.

The origin of *invitation* as my key idea for defining communication of all kinds came from co-teaching in theatre voice classes. At the time, language about vocal volume was framed as "projection" and/or "landing" your voice on the other person. I saw in many of the actors I was teaching (as well as in myself) that when their thinking was about landing their voice on the person opposite them, they further launched their head and whole body toward the other person in a way that caused overall tightening and disturbed breathing.

I first experimented with using the Alexander Technique to carry out the instructions to project the voice. I found that despite clear intentions to use the new plan, the moment of speaking caused discoordination. I also called on F.M. Alexander's story, making sure everyone knew that they had a choice about whether to speak. Still, everyone was generally unsuccessful at sustaining coordination either to project the sound or land their voice on the other people.

As often happens, the moment of failure in teaching caused me to think anew. Recalling my Physics of Music and Speech course from my undergraduate study at Penn State University, I thought, "Right, you can't push sound waves out—all you can do is hang out and resonate." Suddenly, I understood: Sound is not launched! What was happening in these voice classes was that the students were using the Alexander Technique to carry out an impossible plan. They were trying to project sound waves across the room. Since we are biopsychosocially whole, this meant that the Alexander Technique was helping them carry out this impossible plan as well as they could. The plan itself was still impossible, resulting in unnecessary work and tightening between head and spine.

The next step in my investigation: What was it that the students really wanted to do? They needed to generate enough sound waves that the person or people at a distance from them could participate in the story. To accomplish this task, they needed a desire to communicate, as well as knowledge of the size of the space and distance to their audience. (For professional communication that requires a large sound or takes place in a large auditorium, some vocal training is also required.) What the "land the sound on the person you are talking to" instruction was aiming to activate was a desire to communicate over the distance the sound needs to travel. Because much of the voice/speech activation in our systems takes place in the involuntary system, it functions best from "need" to communicate. Consequently, I had to offer the students a plan that would answer the needs of sound production in a way that our design actually could carry out.

I recalled an exercise my director in grad school at Washington University in St. Louis used to help us fill the Edison Theatre. Being heard in Edison was more of a chore than in most theaters. (It was explained that the theater had been designed to work for both spoken word and musical acoustics—and ended up being good for neither. Acoustic modifications have since been made.) While rehearsing Arthur Miller's *Death of a Salesman* in the space, our director, Sid Friedman (the professor who introduced me to Marj), was having trouble hearing us. During the next rehearsal, he asked us to pick a partner. One person stood at the back of the house, while the other stood onstage. Our task was to arrange to meet the other person the next day for lunch. We were shocked to discover how easy it was to get our voice to the back of the auditorium. Sid explained that our success came from having a need, as well as getting more direct feedback about the size of the house, as we could see our partner and knew from their response whether they could hear us.

Investigating further, as I thought about the physics of sound, the gesture of reaching out to someone at a distance, then asking them to come to me appeared—this is what I could do. I could create vibrations with the intent of including people in the vibrational field. Out of these and other investigations, the word *invite* appeared. *Invite* includes need and assumes distance. The gesture of inviting was, in fact, the opposite of the head-launching I observed as people tried to project their sound. When I experimented with asking

TEACHING STORY

During one of our Friday Harbor summer intensives, I wanted to experiment with reciting a poem from memory—an anti-war poem by e.e. cummings ("next to of course god america i") that I, as a literature teacher, knew well and had recited often. First, Cathy had me recite the poem as I saw fit. Then, rather than provide any particular critique or invite it from the group, she asked me to clarify my intentions in sharing the poem with an audience. After some thought, I realized that I wanted to warn listeners about the dangers of crass and unthinking patriotism, as revealed by the poem's speaker. To do that effectively, I had to involve all of my psychophysical self and *become* that speaker. After "making the ask" to allow me to consciously cooperate with myself, I started to recite again—and became someone else. A new kind of feeling entered the room as I paced around making eye contact with each listener, and each line blossomed with deeper and darker implications. Afterward, I found myself running rapidly in place, eager to shake off that creep! Cathy followed up with some very helpful focusing exercises so I could ground myself in the moment, let go of the disturbing emotions, and rejoin the group. Without an Alexander Technique teacher's guidance, I don't believe I would have found my way into—or out of—this depth of performance.

people simply to invite people to the sound they were making, they succeeded in making the appropriate amount of sound—with better quality and fuller resonance and a sustained overall coordination.

Out of what began as an exploration of the coordination of voice grew the realization that *invitation* encompasses my personal communication values while serving a coordination need. In all of my communication, I use the Alexander Technique to invite people to be with me while I am with them.

Invitations are generally associated with pleasant events. Marj's summer flyers were "an invitation to pleasant experiences with the Alexander Technique."

Invitation is kind.

Invitation is honest.

Invitation is respectful.

If teaching is creating the conditions in which someone can learn what they want to learn, then the communication in teaching is an invitation to participate in these conditions. Invitation bolsters freedom of choice; we know that someone can both accept and decline an invitation. Invitation reminds me that as a teacher, I am not in charge of whether someone wants to join in my ideas. All I can do is tailor and reinvent the invitation as needed to incentivize participation.

In the midst of teaching, whenever a person or a group has concerns about a process, I ask myself, "How can I invite this person to this new idea?"

Neuroscience, Relational Field, and Invitation

In addition to the idea of invitation supporting the needs-based regulation of breathing and sound, it also creates the peripersonal and extrapersonal space of the teaching environment. An article in the journal *Cognitive Processing* offers these definitions:

> Peripersonal space is defined as the space immediately surrounding our bodies. Objects within peripersonal space can be grasped and manipulated; objects located beyond this space (in what is often termed "extrapersonal space") cannot normally be reached without moving toward them, or else their movement toward us. (Holmes and Spence 2004, p.94)

In our teaching studios, the peripersonal space describes the field of the students closest to us, and the extrapersonal space encompasses the larger group.

Note that I cite the definition from a reputably scientific source, because, although peripersonal space and extrapersonal space are active research areas, people often seem skeptical about this topic. From the abstract of the same paper:

> In the review that follows, we describe and evaluate recent results from neurophysiology, neuropsychology, and psychophysics in both human and non-human primates that support the existence of an integrated representation of visual, somatosensory, and auditory peripersonal space. Such a representation involves primarily visual, somatosensory, and proprioceptive modalities, operates in body part-centred reference frames, and demonstrates significant plasticity. (Holmes and Spence 2004, p.94)

Sandra and Matthew Blakeslee, writers with an interest in brain science, describe peripersonal space (the musicians) and extrapersonal space (the concert) in experiences familiar to all of us:

> Musicians strive for joint action that transcends each individual. Watch your favorite band in a live jam session. And have you ever gone to a reggae or rock concert where thousands of people move in unison to the music? If you stand back and watch the crowd, you may get a vivid sense of One Big Body Map. Seriously, try it. The same goes for being at a gospel service or for when a batter hits a home run in a baseball stadium. As the crowd leaps to its feet, you can feel the unity of the experience not just in your eyes and ears but in your expanded body map. (Blakeslee and Blakeslee 2007, p.137)

These circumstances are similar to my initial exploration of sound—desire to communicate at a known distance. All that is required is the intention to communicate over the distance you intend. Yes, if it is a very large space, we need to develop some specialized skills for this.

We use the sense of our peripersonal and extrapersonal space all the time—think of the times that you suddenly knew someone was close to you, or how you search for someone in a crowd by thinking of them as you look. As an actor, I was trained to fill the theater, not just with my sound, but with my whole self. Prior to the research regarding extrapersonal space, performing artists have known that when an audience is "with them," the space feels charged. Archie Smith, one of my acting teachers at Penn State, used exercises developed by Michael Chekhov to help us acquire the skills to fill a space—to expand what the Blakeslees call "the bubble around the body" to encompass the whole room (Blakeslee and Blakeslee 2007, p.109). We stood opposite a partner while intending to be with them, then gradually moved farther away. If we sensed that we had lost connection with the other person, we moved closer to reestablish the connection, then challenged ourselves to continue extending it farther away. I now use a larger version of this exercise when I am coaching/directing the company Lucia Neare's Theatrical Wonders. Our large-scale work often takes place outdoors, across immense distances. We need to stay connected over these expanses. We build this ability through practice.

The Teaching Space

I remember a moment, after I had been teaching the Alexander Technique for some years, watching Marj as she moved her hand toward her student. The way I described what I saw to myself was "She is moving in such a way that she doesn't disrupt the field around the student." It was a kind of invisibility—moving and blending with the field so that both participants maintained individual integrity, yet shared their field. From that day, I chose to add this to my intent in teaching: "How do I move in such a way that I respect this person's field?"

The burgeoning field of neuroscience continues to gather evidence on how we communicate. Recently, researchers from the University College London Division of Psychological and Language Sciences "monitored the heart rates and electro dermal activity of 12 audience members at a live performance of the West End musical *Dreamgirls*. The team found that the audience members' hearts were responding in unison, with their pulses speeding up and slowing down at the same rate." From Dr Joe Devlin, who led the study:

> Usually, a group of individuals will each have their own heart rates and rhythms, with little relationship to each other. But romantic couples or highly effective teammates will actually synchronise their hearts so that they beat in time with each other, which in itself is astounding… This clearly demonstrates that the physiological synchrony observed

during the performance was strong enough to overcome social group differences and engage the audience as a whole. (University College London Psychology and Language Sciences 2017)

Although I lack data, my experience is that using the Alexander Technique to invite people to be with you while you are with them facilitates the same "withing" experience these scientists are investigating.

When an Idea Doesn't Work

Another metaphor I use to describe my teaching communication is that I am walking with my students in their process. This leaps to my attention, particularly when an interaction goes in some way awry in the teaching room.

The Cathy Glossary in Chapter 2 introduces "back-pocket plan." I have made such plans for myself for the moments in a lesson when communication difficulties occur:

> I ask myself to COORDINATE so that my head can move so that all of me can follow so that, knowing that everything that happens in a teaching space is somehow about the learning process, I can gather information so that I will know what I want to do.

In this case, the back-pocket plan includes renewal of knowledge I already have—"knowing that everything that happens in a teaching space is somehow about the learning process." Renewing this knowing takes care of any concern or fear I might have if a student doesn't understand, while calling up any information that might be useful in the lesson itself. If the nature of the response is emotional, then I might also renew the knowledge—for myself, the student, and the group—that emotions are natural and safe.

My pledge is to walk with my students through these moments. Most of the time, we sort things out; if not that day, then another. Some interactions and the occasional impasse do reveal that we genuinely have different beliefs, which I would say is what we both need to know. Sometimes, miscommunication comes about when a bit of humor or the way I say something unexpectedly creates a condition in which they are angry, or frightened, or feel judged. I trust that anything that happens in the learning playground is related to how someone needs to learn. Using the AT Progression, I walk with my student's emotional response, assuring goodwill and restoring a constructive learning environment.

Store Clerk Practice

I use what I call "Store Clerk Practice" myself and offer it to my students. When experimenting with new ideas in communication, I use the Alexander Technique to practice with store clerks, baristas, bus drivers—whomever I encounter in my daily life. Because these are often people I would see only once or perhaps a few times, the consequences of failure are not significant, giving me a safe playground to experiment with any ideas that seem on my edge of comfort. Since all of my intentions in communication are intended kindly, the store clerk is not at risk. I note that this practice usually seems to be received well, perhaps by personalizing the encounter enough to add a little warmth to an everyday moment.

Chapter 7

HAVING A "YES" PLAN

As I sift through memories of my sometimes-excruciating exercises in my Meisner-based first acting class at Penn State, I recognize that in the made-up scenarios, success occurred when I said "yes" to pursuing what I wanted rather than dwelling on trying to feel or illustrate the scenario. The story was revealed through the "yes" of my pursuit. (The Meisner Technique focuses on actor preparation and on listening and responding precisely to your scene partners.)

Yes takes wants into action. In theatre, the imagined scenarios include obstacles because theatre needs a conflict to be dramatic. The obstacle could be considered a "no" in relationship to what the actor and/or character wants in the scene. Acting goes awry when the actor plays the obstacle rather than the action, the "no" rather than the "yes." Out of my experience, I have always coached acting from the perspective of *want* and *yes*, a practice reinforced by my Alexander Technique-based omniservations.

A significant moment in my getting to "yes" occurred in Marj's house. When she was out of town, she had me open the curtains and turn off the lights in the morning, and vice versa in the evening. Being in your teacher's house is an excellent cue for utilizing what she is teaching you. So, I decided to ask myself to COORDINATE so that my head could move so that all of me could follow so that I could lead with my fingers to reach for every lamp and curtain. I would sometimes step back and redo the process if I thought I had tightened between head and spine.

One day, I realized that every time I stopped, I tightened to stop—and I tightened to notice what I was doing. My questions to myself were "Do I need to tighten more to start using the Alexander Technique?" "Do I need to tighten to notice what I am doing?" I hoped the answer was "no" and devised a new experiment. I wondered what would happen if, when I thought I had tightened unnecessarily in reaching for a lamp, rather than stopping and saying "no" to myself, I could simply say "yes" by asking myself to do what I wanted to do— "to send a wish to my head and spine so that all of me could follow so that I could reach for the lamp." I didn't have to know whether I had tightened—I could simply use the Alexander Technique and continue turning the lamp on or off. I repeated my experiment many times while moving curtains and flicking light switches. Ultimately, I realized I was reaching for objects in the rest of my daily life with a "yes" plan. I found that I could omniserve and make new plans for myself in action.

When I coached the Alexander Technique during a camera acting class, what appeared through the camera's viewfinder reaffirmed that such a constructive emphasis in the Alexander Technique—the "yes" to the new idea—is vital. The swiftness with which any thought involving a "no," "not," or "don't" caused an actor to stiffen was remarkable. On film, such excessive muscular work causes the actor to lose the subtle facial and eye movement that reveals the character and story. The camera acting teacher and I discovered this in class when reviewing what we had just filmed, both of us singling out a particular moment as one where something had gone wrong—the camera "didn't like her," and we couldn't follow her story. Knowing she had tightened between head and spine at that moment, I asked her what she had been thinking, which was "I don't want to listen to my scene partner." Although her analysis of the script correctly identified that she wasn't listening to the other character, she hadn't gone the next step to figure out what she was listening to. This negative thought—"I don't want to listen"— immediately caused her overall tightening, particularly involving the face and eye muscles, creating a static rather than dynamic relationship between actor and camera. We replaced her acting thought with what she wanted, with her "yes"—"I would like to be listening to a song." She remained in coordination, the camera "liked" her, and the story was served because, indeed, she looked like she wasn't listening to him.

Daniel Siegel's work in the field of interpersonal neurobiology embraces "yes." In his procedure of alternating saying "no" and "yes," he finds that "'no' evokes these reactions to threat; 'yes' often relaxes this reactivity and enables us to enter a state of receptivity" (Siegel 2012, p.18-4).

Back in the world of the theatre, Second City members Leonard and Yorton note the power of *yes and*: "These two words form the bedrock of all improvisation… This simple idea has amazing power and potency to improve interpersonal communication, negotiation, and conflict resolution" (2015, p.13).

I discuss the power of word choice more thoroughly in a later chapter. Note here that committing to a "yes" plan requires ongoing considered word selection. I have made it my daily practice to speak exactingly from the perspective of "yes."

TEACHING STORY

I was playing my cello in a workshop, and feeling some pressure. Cathy asked about my intention. I replied that I wanted to make my audience feel sad. Cathy pointed out that I have no control over how other people feel, and that the tension came from trying to do something impossible. She suggested I merely invite the audience to come along with me on my musical journey. When I did that, the pressure vanished and my coordination improved. I have been inviting audiences to come along with me ever since.

Chapter 8

OMNISERVATION

"How did you see that?" "What are you seeing?" "How did you know what to ask about in that moment?" These are perhaps the questions I receive most often when teaching continuing education workshops for Alexander Technique teachers. As I mentioned in Chapter 1, while the questions are usually framed visually, they really address how I am receiving information through all of my senses, hence my evolution from *observation* to *omniservation*.

By "all my senses," I mean many more than the five that most of us were taught to identify. In 2005, *The New Scientist* published a chart listing 10 conservatively accepted senses, 21 accepted senses, and 33 that were considered radical. Here is the "accepted" list: light, color, hearing, smell (2000 or more receptor types), taste (sweet, salt, sour, bitter, umami), touch, pain, balance, proprioception, kinaesthesis, heat, cold, blood pressure, blood oxygen content, cerebrospinal fluid pH, thirst and hunger (Durie 2005, p.34).

How I Developed Omniservation

So far, the information I have offered on how I developed these skills are:

- Marj's Living Room Étude: If I wanted to be able to teach, I needed to be able to say what I saw.

- Acting and directing training—they require the same skills.

- Commitment to giving words to omniservation, resulting in increased confidence.

In addition, I studied dance for many years. Part of that training is to be able to watch a movement and immediately replicate it.

Other factors that have developed my omniservation skills, specifically for Alexander Technique teaching:

- I watched people who do things well who don't know the Alexander Technique. I still do this, calling it "keeping my eyes honest."

- I omniserve the role of geometry and physics relative to movement.

- I stopped trying to teach the lesson before I omniserved.

- Along the way, I lost my fear of omniserving "wrong." I realized that if I state something inaccurately, the student usually corrects me, and then we have the information we need. The objective isn't about whether I am right, but about the student having what they need to learn what they want to learn.

- I continue to refine my knowledge of human movement and behavior by studying anatomy and physiology, psychology, linguistics, neuroscience of various kinds, and other relevant subjects.

- Practice. Along with commitment to naming what I experience.

Developing the Skill

One of my strong memories of my first workshop with Marj in Nebraska was sitting in the large group thinking, "What on earth are they seeing?" Over the next weeks and months, I took Marj's advice simply to wonder about what I was watching. When people asked her what she was seeing, I had the opportunity to correlate what I had noticed with what she or someone else reported. Over time, these skills "came online." When I informally take learning preferences tests, I don't test high in the visual category. This is to say, I had to learn to omniserve—it wasn't an overnight event. It takes practice.

100 Days, a solo dance performed and choreographed by Peter Kyle, "built entirely from borrowed movements gathered over 100 days of studying 100 everyday people as they moved about their lives"

(Kyle 2012), is informative and inspiring as to the amount of detail it is possible to omniserve.

Some years ago, when I was considering how to confront any bias I might have about ideal coordination, omniserving people who do things well who don't know the Alexander Technique was one of my chosen tasks. Successful athletes were the easiest to track over time. Most elite athletes move very well. Even the ones who don't move as well proved valuable to study—they tend to get injured more often because they are compensating for their lack of optimal coordination with less appropriate muscle action. Athletes are also frequently interviewed after their performances, sometimes even before performances, which gives me information about how their thinking informs what I am about to see or just saw. Performing artists were also included in this query.

> **TEACHING STORY**
>
> In one of my first lessons with Cathy, I wanted her to help me sing. Instead of instructing me to get "it" away from my lips, or relax my jaw, as previous teachers had told me, she asked me if I used to play the flute. "Yes!" I cried, amazed, and sure that she was psychic. "It looks like you are trying to adjust your lips to a flute, or trying to form an embouchure that is right for the flute, but not for singing." Cathy happened to have a flute on hand. She observed what I did with my mouth as I played it. We then talked about the differences required for playing the flute and singing. I played. I sang. It was a revelation.

They were not, however, as available on a continual basis to watch. And, while they may write or be interviewed about their craft, artist interviews are more often reflective rather than in-the-moment reports. (Wouldn't it be interesting to have pre- and post-show interview reporters backstage?)

I call all of this omniservational practice "keeping my eyes honest." It is a daily practice for me that continues to contribute to my skills at analyzing activity, the continual study of practical anatomy.

Solo Practice Idea–Anywhere, Anytime

When people ask me how to teach themselves this skill, I offer a series of omniservation experiments. This series is based on my best reconstruction of my own sequence in learning to omniserve. Watching passersby walking down the street, watching the barista make your cappuccino, watching sports, watching a class through the window of a dance studio, watching teenagers walking to school, watching children in the playground, watching people pump their gas—the possibilities are endless. It can be helpful to watch people on video doing various things, though the speed and nonrepeatability of live practice are more like the real teaching moment. I recommend staying with each practice long enough to gain confidence in carrying the skill forward to the next practice.

First Practice

Observe what they are doing, so you can describe exactly what you see. You aren't necessarily thinking about the quality of the activity. Simply ask yourself, "What are they actually doing?"

Second Practice

Next, add the question, "What do I notice in the relationship between their head and spine as they are doing what they are doing?" Ask yourself to describe this in as much detail as possible.

Third Practice

Add the question, "How does what they are doing in their head–spine relationship relate to what is happening in the rest of them? How does it relate to their activity?"

Fourth Practice

Add the question, "What might make it perfect that this is the way they are doing what they are doing?" You won't be able to ask questions to verify your guesses; rather, you are practicing curiosity, deepening your understanding that people always make perfect choices based on the information they have.

Your guesses may or may not be accurate. While guessing is something we will do, in life and in teaching, we don't want to assume we are accurate. I voice very few of my guesses when teaching; when I do venture a guess, it goes something like, "I don't know what you are thinking, but if I guessed…" Or, "This is a guess, but do you have the idea…?" For me, owning guesses is vital in communication; I do not want to impose my perception on my student. Having taught many people who have been affected adversely by someone's label or interpretation, I clearly identify guesses as guesses.

Fifth Practice

Follow the sequence of the previous practices, beginning with accuracy of omniservation, and wonder what question you might ask this person if you could.

Sixth Practice

Follow the sequence of the previous practices, beginning with accuracy of omniservation, and wonder what constructive plan you might offer.

For me, the active curiosity these practices promote helps me appreciate the richness of people's choices in daily life. Although I have offered these for solo practice, groups can use them as well. Once a whole workshop bundled up in our coats and walked to a dock to embark on a slightly windy boat tour. We omniserved our fellow passengers and discreetly compared notes.

I Omniserve, I Wonder, I Perceive

Richard Nichols taught me this exercise adapted from Eric Morris's acting exercises (Morris and Hotchkis 2002[1977], p.50). In the acting exercise, you have a partner who can hear what you are saying. For the purposes of Alexander Technique teaching, you could do the exercise for many of the situations that introduced the practices—just silently.

While you are watching someone, fill in these blanks:

I omniserve _____

I wonder _____

I perceive _____

Wonder is a call to curiosity, perhaps the beginning of a question. *Perceive* often needs explanation. It can mean interpret, or become conscious of something. It is, like the Third Practice above, a way of asking yourself to acknowledge what the omniservation and wonder have brought up for you. How are you interpreting these? "I perceive" is another way to note what your assumptions and guesses are.

This is also a tool you can use actively while teaching. For example, I omniserve that the student tightened between head and spine in a way that put a concave shape in his thoracic and lumbar spine as he told me about how lifting weights was going well and he'd like to work on speaking; I wonder if this particular pattern is revealing something about the weight lifting; I perceive that I have a guess that there is something in his weight lifting that I might ask about, if it appears germane, after or during our experimentation with speaking.

All of my studies and practices in omniservation are intended to build more tools for teaching. Delicately insist on giving words to what you're omniserving, striving to be as precise and accurate as possible, knowing there is always more to learn.

Chapter 9

ANALYSIS OF ACTIVITY

Omniservation opens up the world of analysis of activity. Not only what am I omniserving, but what is the order and intent of the sequence of actions I am witnessing?

Analysis of Activity Sequence

Table 9.1 shows the primary questions that guide me as I analyze what my student is doing.

Table 9.1 Analysis of Activity

What exactly are they doing? In what sequence are they doing it?	
How would I describe their coordination while they do it? What is happening between head and spine? What makes how it is happening perfect?	
What do I know, if anything, about the activity, skill, or question they have? Have I done it myself? Have I taught anyone else who does this or something like it?	
What do I know about human design that might contribute to the student's question or request?	
Do I know any resources that might be helpful? Are they available?	

What Exactly Are They Doing? In What Sequence Are They Doing It?

A trumpet player came to me for a lesson. As I watched him play, I was mystified. I could, of course, see certain things, but much of what I was watching was new to me. Fortunately, I could enlist the musician's aid. I omniserved as much as I could, then asked questions to gather more information, such as, "What do you need to do to use your air the way you want to?" and "If you were teaching someone how to play in the higher registers, how would you explain this?" Later, I also watched videos of a trumpeter whom my student had identified as highly skilled.

A Word about "Exactly"

Striving to be as precise as possible, as noted at the end of the Omniservation chapter, is a life-long task. This is why I coach teachers first to omniserve what is happening right in the moment of

> **TEACHING STORY**
> In an intensive, a lot of us came with questions about arm structure and arm movements. Arm movements became a recurring theme of the workshop. You asked us each to think of an activity involving arm movements—something we had a lot of experience with—and then you asked us to teach some of the movements to the other students there. One person played the piano, another person did some swimming, another cut vegetables with a knife, and so on. In order to teach these movements to the others, we each had to work out what exactly we were doing ourselves. Often, we created what we thought were clear instructions, only to realize that when the others faithfully followed our words, they couldn't perform the activity. We realized that the instructions themselves were unclear or had gaps, which prompted us to elaborate and clarify our plan for the activity. I learned a lot about all kinds of arm movements, not least in the activity I thought I already knew best!

teaching before developing a teaching idea/plan. What does this particular person mink and thove to accomplish the task? Even if you have seen another person engaged in the same activity, each person has a unique approach.

In a break from writing this book, I watched the ISU Grand Prix of Figure Skating. Analyzing how different ice-dancing pairs accomplished similar lifts, spins, and step sequences was fascinating. Because the skaters were all different sizes in relationship to one another, the way in which each pair designed their version of particular skills was necessarily unique to them. How their heads moved to flow with and/or counterbalance a move was an anatomy/physics/geometry puzzle. Hearing the commentator explain why something worked or didn't work supplemented my omniservation.

Every pianist has a different mechanical advantage in relationship to the piano; every computer set-up is different, so the way in which people move to type is different; some shoes require a new organization to support coordination. Seeing what is specific to each individual matters, because accurate feedback drives learning in each unique teaching moment.

I omniserve and I ask. I am not the expert on what my students are doing—they are. As I teach them, I often do research on activities new to me, yet my role remains in service to the *how* of what they are doing. What I love is that by inviting students directly to COORDINATE *to do what they are doing*, we get immediate feedback on whether the new Alexander Technique plan works. The experiment is an immediate litmus test, the canary in the coal tunnel that lets me know if what I have offered is actually utilitarian. Such immediate application keeps the Alexander Technique practical, based in life rather than in theory.

How Would I Describe Their Coordination while They Do It? What Is Happening between Head and Spine? What Makes How It Is Happening Perfect?

With a clearer picture of what students are doing and/or intend to be doing, I watch carefully to see when they are sustaining a cooperating coordination, and note when something seems out of place. Often, the student gives me a clue about when to look for a change in coordination, such as, "When I dribble the basketball around the court, my legs seem to be moving well. After I take a shot at the basket, I have trouble starting to move again." Clearly, I am going to be watching what happens at the moment the student identified. Not only that moment, however: sometimes, what happens at that particular moment occurs because of something that preceded it. I avidly accept all offered clues, while gathering my own as well.

Always, always, always, I remind myself that what is happening is perfect in some way. If I listen carefully, I might hear how someone is phrasing a step in their activity that doesn't meet the criteria for a change plan. The result they are getting is perfect relative to what they are asking for; what needs to change is what they are asking for, the plan for the activity itself. Perhaps, for instance, this imagined basketball player had been given the idea to ground himself before taking a shot, and mistakenly carried out the idea of grounding by tightening the legs and feet to *feel* grounded. That would explain the problem. I could offer a plan to replace the idea of grounding with my plan for standing, something like:

> Ask yourself to COORDINATE so that your head can move so that all of you can follow so that you can run to the spot you want, put your right foot somewhere and your left foot somewhere, knowing you can go anywhere any time, so that you can move the ball in the direction you want, ready to move your legs in a new direction of travel.

Fortunately, "think speed" is much faster than "speak speed." My key would be the word *grounded* that potentially matched the tightening the student described. I would need to help the student redefine grounding and identify what the task actually required.

I think of a professional ballet dancer. He was obviously quite good, but started to tighten between head and spine as he moved his arms to prepare to dance. We tried using the Alexander Technique to make the arm movement and the same thing happened. Because of the timing of his tightening, I asked a question about how he thought of his arms. We uncovered a message from when he was little boy learning to dance and someone told him to make his arms round. He was still doing that, really trying to do that, which is impossible. What he described matched what we were seeing—you could see his muscles working hard to bend bones that were essentially straight. When he used the Alexander Technique to use his arms to, instead, create the illusion of a curving arm, the whole group gasped as we experienced the new quality of his movement.

What Do I Know, if Anything, about the Activity, Skill, or Question They Have? Have I Done It Myself? Have I Taught Anyone Else Who Does This or Something Like It?

In the examples of activities I have chosen so far—trumpet, piano, basketball, ice skating, dancing—the only one I have studied personally is dancing. I have taught myself some piano, I have fooled around with a basketball, I have loved watching ice skating since I was a child, though the only time I was on ice skates was when I was a camp counselor at Camp Akiba and I had to pretend I knew what I was doing to keep my eight-year-old charges skating. I have at least held a trumpet.

Alexander Technique teachers are gifted with glimpses into new worlds of experience. Performing artists, computer programmers, engineers, athletes, and people from many walks of life with many avocations have told me how they think about what they are doing. My dean at the university once asked me to list activities I had taught Alexander Technique in relationship to them. The partial list I wrote includes:

> Acting/Directing; Circus Skills; Communication (Speaking/ Listening/Counseling); Computer/Office Ergonomics; Dancing (Ballet, Modern, Jazz, Lindy Hop, Salsa, Swing, Tap, Clogging); Drafting; Decision-Making; Household Tasks; Lighting Design; Massage; Meditation; Movement Training (Pilates, Yoga, etc.); Musicians (Accordion, Bass, Clarinet, Conducting, French Horn, Guitar, Harp, Oboe, Organ, Percussion, Piano, Piccolo, Trombone, Trumpet, Violin, Viola); Post-Traumatic Stress Disorder (aid to changing response patterns once psychiatric needs have been taken care of); Pottery; Public Speaking; Sales Training; Singing (Classical, Musical Comedy, Jazz, Pop); Sports (Baseball, Bicycling, Bowling, Cricket, Discus, Dressage, Football, Golf, Rock Climbing, Rowing, Running/Jogging, Tennis, Track Cycling, Weight Lifting); Translating (helping translators with their coordination as they translate); Visual Arts (Painting, Photography, Sculpting); Writing.

Each time I analyze a new skill, my teaching vocabulary grows. My students have increased my vocabulary immensely. At the moment of omniserving, I am using the Alexander Technique to invite my whole self to provide any information that can fuel the teaching, and am prepared to ask, "I don't know what you need to do. Can you describe it to me?"

What Do I Know about Human Design That Might Contribute to This Request?

Anatomy, physiology, psychology, and neuroscience offer worlds of new information. Alexander Technique teachers are lucky because our job always invites us to learn more and more and more...

Do I Know Any Resources That Might Be Helpful? Are They Available?

My studio has a lot of resources for anatomy/physiology. I like actually pulling out a picture or a resource as I discuss an anatomical question so that I can assure, as much as possible, an accurate understanding. After viewing the resource, we move, using the new information in dimensional space. This also keeps me learning. If I am away from those resources, my own body serves as an anatomy guide. With some activities, I will do research between lessons.

Step by Step in Activities of Your Choice

Analyzing your own activities is another way to build your skills. If I were to pick up my teacup right now, here is one version of how I could break down that activity into component steps:

> Using the Alexander Technique, I
>
> Move my eyes to the left.
>
> Tilt my head down and to the left to see my cup.
>
> Flex at the elbow joint slightly to take fingers off of computer keyboard.
>
> Externally rotate at the gleno-humeral joint so my fingers are over the cup. (I am standing, by the way.)
>
> Extend at the elbow joint as my fingers lead to the rim of the cup in such a way that my fingers can move in the shape of the cup.
>
> Slide my fingers slightly backwards to move around the handle of the cup, noting this involves a slight roll backward in the gleno-humeral joint.
>
> Flex my elbow joint and internally rotate at the gleno-humeral joint, with slight motion at the sterno-clavicular joint as I move the cup to my mouth.
>
> Move slightly at the glenohumeral joint and wrist joints, with slight rocking at the sterno-claivicular joint to tilt the cup so that the tea goes into my mouth, noting that as I do that, my thumb is counterbalancing the tea cup.

I could go into further detail—for instance, about the angles of the fingers and wrist as I pick up the cup—and I might need to if my student's question has to do with wrist or finger pain/restriction. As you explore these yourself in a variety of activities, your ability to analyze activities in your students will increase.

Chapter 10

TACTILE COMMUNICATION

My refined, subtle, flexible skill to use my hands as part of whole-self communication in teaching the Alexander Technique developed in Marj's living room. We'd ask Marj how to do it and heard, "If you are interested in how to use your hands as part of the teaching process, pay attention to what you do with them all day." Consequently, many of us asked for lessons on daily tasks that used our hands: picking up books off of the floor, turning on lights, drinking a cup of tea, moving the arms in a dance movement, and so on. In these turns, Marj was meticulous—first about our overall coordination, then about the particulars of the arm movement. The consistent instructions I remember are "Let your fingers lead to the object," "Let the object shape your hand," and "Look at your hand." (*Note*: Rather than *let*, I have changed to using active verbs in my own version of teaching students how to use their hands to do things.)

Learning to Use My Hands to Teach

One day, I heard her say once again, "If you are interested in how to use your hands as part of the teaching process, pay attention to what you do with them all day." And I thought, "She means that." From that day on, I decided that every time I used my hands, I wanted to let my fingers lead to the object, let the object shape my hand, and look at what I was doing. Reaching for something became an external cue for me to use the Alexander Technique. When Charles Duhigg talks about changing behavior in his book *The Power of Habit*, he says:

The process within our brains is a three-step loop. First, there is a *cue,* a trigger that tells your brain to go into the automatic mode and which habit to use. Then there is the *routine,* which can be physical, mental or emotional. Finally, there is the *reward,* which helps your brain figure out if this particular loop is worth remembering for the future... (Duhigg 2012, p.19; original emphasis)

In my book on using the Alexander Technique for performance, I rewrote his phrase in relationship to the conscious process of the Alexander Technique:

In learning to use the Alexander Technique for performance, and to cooperate with how we are designed to learn, it is useful to have an external cue (a cue from something in your activity or environment rather than just something you directly notice about yourself) to signal to yourself that you want to use the AT. The Alexander Technique plan is the *process.* The *reward* appears either immediately or over time in the continued improvement in your coordination and your ability to use same in service of your desires. (Madden 2014, p.272)

While my commitment to reaching for everything using the Alexander Technique predated Duhigg's research, I was clearly using an external cue to learn how to use my hands for everything, including teaching. I even remember dancing and watching my hands the whole time—fingers leading in the air. This practice remains part of my daily life.

Through this continued practice, skilled touch and a high quality of coordination in relationship to using my hands was available to me by the time I was ready to teach. As noted earlier, the first time I got close enough to my student to use my hands as part of my communication, I seemed to know what to do. With the precision of my omniservation and the studied rehearsed plan for moving my hands and arms, I understood how my hands could assist in the communication process. Consistently using my hands constructively as part of the teaching process took time, but the idea that my hands were making a request of the student—asking—appeared early in my teaching career.

A significant lesson that shaped my understanding of tactile communication occurred in one of Marj's quick walk sessions. We were in a line, each waiting for our turn. She interrupted what she was doing to say, "You know, you don't have to wait to 'ask to ease' until you get to me. You can be talking to yourself already." Having learned by then that if she said something, she probably meant it, I started to use the Alexander Technique while waiting; and then, when my quick turn began, she joined in the process I had already begun. What I was able to learn from her when already in process myself was profound.

Consequently, from that day on, I endeavored to be *already in process* as my lesson with Marj began. As I emphasize when I discuss the introductory lesson in a later chapter, I now choose to give that responsibility to my students from their first lesson, communicating from the get-go, "The primary use of my hands in teaching is to follow you as you change as a 'yes' to the new idea."

Marj was adamant that we watch our hands as we moved them toward our student. Her explanation was that we would see the quality with which we were moving and be able to adjust as needed. I add to this explanation that if you are watching your hands, you also see what the student is doing and can adjust to them as well. Her suggested practice is sound science: Berthoz emphasizes in *The Brain's Sense of Movement* that movement requires multisensory input: "These data suggest that tactile inputs have access to the centers of the brain that process visual information… These two modalities are also involved in the coherent perception of one's own body and in establishing multiple frames of reference to different parts of the body" (2000, p.85). Marj also would frequently tell us during our lessons to actually look at what we were doing; she didn't mean this metaphorically, but concretely. We can see most of ourselves as we are moving, and watching the movement helps recalibrate new ideas. Combining vision with movement and tactile input is deep training for the self.

> **TEACHING STORY**
> It was the last day of a ten-day workshop, and I was a little exhausted. So, as Cathy was explaining something while making her rounds with her exquisite and effectful "hands on," I was happily expecting my turn, already "relaxing." But she saw me and said, "Oh look, she is expecting me to do the work"—and crossed the room to the other side of the people's circle! First I was very upset! and immediately knew that sitting is an activity…and my head started leading, everything following…and I got the feedback "sitting like a queen on her throne" from the other participants.

My articulation of how I describe using my hands in teaching continues to evolve over time. Choosing to use my hands to follow my students as they change as a "yes" to the new idea is congruent with many of my values:

- Just as in the quick turn lesson I had with Marj, I want my students to be the ones in charge of "the ask." As I explain to them, "I can follow you as you change as a 'yes' to the new idea; what I can't do is 'ask'—that is your job."

- Each person restores to their own coordination uniquely. With the omniservation skills I learned from Marj, I can watch what is happening so that I respond in the use of my hands to each individual's process and structure.

- I also describe using my hands in relationship to knowing that all patterns are perfect. "It seems to help if I use my hands to follow you as you change as a 'yes' to the new idea. However you have been moving has been perfect in some way. As you start to respond to your ask, sometimes that old perfect idea jumps in and says, 'Wait, you forgot me!' When I use my hands to follow the change you are asking for, it helps you stay with the new idea longer."

- Omniservation of my student helps me to use my hands only until it looks like the student is ready to move with the new idea on their own. We are moving on the edge of the learning frontier—seeking the area in which the challenge is reachable and ultimately sustainable.

My choice to follow my students as they change grew out of somewhat of a career crisis at the International Congress of Alexander Technique in Engelberg, Switzerland, in 1991. I spent one afternoon moving from room to room, spending five to ten minutes in many sessions. My impression was that in every room (except one in which the teacher was speaking tangentially), people were saying virtually the same thing. How they moved, however, didn't match what I would expect—each group's manifestation of what they were saying looked different from the other groups. My sense of truth, cultivated from theatre training, sounded an alarm. If we are well designed, and if the intention of the Alexander Technique is either to replace any interference or preserve coordinated responses in our biopsychosocial selves, then I didn't think we should look so differently room to room. Knowing that I needed to begin with an investigation of my own bias, I set out to explore my concerns. Because how I use my hands to communicate when teaching the work emerged from how I worked through this inquiry, I offer here a summary of my investigation:

- I named the differences I omniserved "Alexander aesthetics," rather than labeling them right or wrong.

- I challenged myself to reexamine my beliefs and biases by...

  - Omniserving people who do things well and don't know the Alexander Technique.

  - Continuing to study how humans move, think, and coordinate.

  - Examining other models of teaching.

  - Clarifying my own teaching process.

My working question was "How can I teach in such a way that the Alexander Technique process sustains and—if necessary—restores cooperation with our natural design in service of what we do?"

Returning to my teaching studio, I renewed and strengthened my commitment to affirming my students as the leaders in their own learning process. Their choices and thinking initiated the process. When I chose to use my hands as part of the teaching process, I was as meticulous as possible in "following them as they change as a 'yes' to the new idea." Although these are not the words Marj used, she taught me the skills I needed to follow through with my choice. The questions arising from my experience at the Congress challenged me to articulate clearly how I used my hands in teaching. Moreover, this also led to my renewed recognition that F.M. Alexander's formulation of the work required that the "Alexander ask" be inclusive of the activity, as in my current phraseology: "What happens if you ask yourself to COORDINATE so that your head can move so that all of you can follow *so that you can do what you are doing?*"

As we all must do, I continue to develop the quality of my use of my hands as part of the teaching process. As Marj taught me, I use the Alexander Technique to lead with my fingertips, looking at my hands as I move toward my student (meaning that I also see my student), then moving my hands in such a way that my fingers move in the shape of the person I am teaching.

The last phrase, "then moving my hands in such a way that my fingers move in the shape of the person I am teaching," is a revision of what I learned from Marj. I have made the phrasing more active— "moving my hands/fingers"—rather than the more passive, "letting my fingers move." I choose the more active language now out of concern that passive language choices in teaching disempower students.

Here is a more complete version of my volitional thinking in relationship to the use of my hands in teaching:

> I ask myself to COORDINATE so that my head can move
> so that all of me can follow
> so that I can invite my student to be with me while I am with them
> so that I can move my fingers toward the student
> so that my fingers/hands move in the shape of the person I am teaching
> so that I can ask them to ask themselves to COORDINATE
> so that their head can move
> so that all of them can follow
> so that they can do what they are doing,
> so that I can follow them as they change as a "yes" to the new idea.

My skill in using my hands this way is also an element of my intent to move invisibly in my students' fields.

Precision Skills in Using One's Hands to Teach

Following are contributing ideas, impressions, and clarifications of some of the many factors that contribute to the effectiveness of tactile communication in teaching the Alexander Technique.

Using My Hands Is about Asking

Occasionally, someone asks me what I am trying to feel when I am using my hands to teach. I have no answer for them—I use my hands to follow the student's coordinating movement as they rediscover their design. While I don't ignore information I may receive tactilely, my sole intent is to ask. Any information that arrives via the feeling senses has the characteristics of all sensory feedback: it is comparative, it is a report of the past, and it reports capriciously. In this instance, it is also unclear whether what I am feeling is about me or about my student. I use my hands to ask.

Choice and Permission

People need to know that they have a choice about the use of touch in the lesson. Touch is just one of many tools we use in teaching. I assure each introductory group that everyone is free to choose at any time whether I use my hands in teaching.

Where Do I Put My Hands?

Marj never answered this question, and for the most part neither do I. Deciding where and how to use your hands to communicate comes as a result of omniservation and analysis. And because no matter where I use my hands in teaching, I am talking whole self to whole self—I am always asking the whole person.

When introducing the Alexander Technique, I tend to use my hands in what I might describe as a logical sequence. My Alexander Technique process is a sequential one that begins with the head–spine relationship. Because this is new information for most people, using my hands first near the head and spine helps reorient them to a whole-self ask rather than a parts-oriented ask. In one workshop, we named this ask "calling whole self via head and spine" so that you can do what you are doing.

When asked this question, I often demonstrate by asking someone if I am able to "ask whole" by touching them somewhere less logical, perhaps with one finger on their little finger or elbow. They discover that I am still communicating whole. Occasionally, it is useful to use my hands far away from the source of the interference: Sometimes, someone is ticklish; sometimes, a particular spot is sensitized by past trauma; sometimes, particularly if someone is moving around a lot, I am simply finding the most convenient spot. No matter where I choose to use my hands, I am guided by "How do I create the conditions in which my students can learn what they want to learn?"

Primary, Not Only

I am meticulous about teaching my students to use the Alexander Technique on their own before using my hands as part of the teaching process. I cannot follow them as they change as a "yes" to the new idea unless they are already asking to COORDINATE so that they can do what they are doing. While, of course, they refine their skills over time, they are from the start the leaders of their own process.

I tell my students, "I primarily use my hands to follow you as you change, and I might use them in other ways, too. Sometimes I might guide a movement—or just get in your way. Very rarely, you might experience what I call an elevator ride. In all cases I am asking you to ask yourself to use the Alexander Technique to do what you are doing." Although I don't have a strict rule about when or if I might make these choices, my intention is always to wait until the students understand their responsibility in the process.

To reiterate my process of using my hands in teaching, because it is vital:

> I ask myself to COORDINATE so that my head can move
> so that all of me can follow
> so that I can invite my student to be with me while I am with them
> so that I can move my fingers toward the student
> so that my fingers/hands move in the shape of the person I am teaching
> so that I can ask them to ask themselves to COORDINATE
> so that their head can move
> so that all of them can follow
> so that they can do what they are doing*
> so that I can follow them as they change as a 'yes' to the new idea.

The asterisk indicates a possible timing/place for alternate uses of touch in teaching, which might include the following.

Guiding Movement

This is most often related to anatomy. Perhaps the student is making a movement and learning where the joints actually are, or discovering a pathway for movement they didn't know existed. I think of this as somewhat akin to the people who guide airplanes to the gate—I am guiding them in the new pathway. What is key is that the student is still the one doing the muscular action. Every so often, someone tries to "give" me their arm or leg, and I complain that I am too lazy for that. They need to participate.

Creating the Conditions for Information

Sometimes, someone has a strong pattern that is so familiar to them, they can't conceive of moving without it. I think of a young man who must have taught himself to tighten his biceps before doing anything (probably a teenage conception). He became so used to this that he didn't know he did it. To help him realize what he was doing so that he could consider another choice, I needed to create the conditions in which he perceived what he was doing. In this kind of situation, I coordinate myself to use as much force as the student is using— possibly a bit more than they are using—to match the pressure of the tightening pattern—just enough that the student can perceive how they are getting in their own way: "Oh, I am tightening my bicep before I do everything!" With the particular student I am recalling, he was tightening so much that I couldn't match his power; and he remained quite sure he wasn't pressing his arms down as I described. I recruited another class member—his workout partner—and coached him on what I was doing. It was a funny moment: as he started to move, his workout partner matched the unhelpful tightening, then stopped and said, "Dude, you are pushing your arms down." "I'm not!" "YOU ARE!" What was lovely about the interchange was that it enabled the inveterate bicep tightener, whose sense of humor rose to the occasion, to reexamine his choices, and the fluidity that appeared in his movement was astounding.

Getting in the Way

When I "get in the way," I coordinate myself to match the pressure of the interfering pattern, then just wait to see if the student can figure out what to do with this information. (Always ready to follow them instantly as they figure it out!) For example, if someone's usual plan for starting to walk involves leaning to one side, I might lightly use my hands on that side so that they notice they are leaning in that direction. In noticing this, they have an opportunity to make a new decision—perhaps to go forward rather than to the side. With experienced students, this can be a funny moment because—for a moment—it seems like you cannot move. Using my hands this way provides a puzzle for the student to work out for themselves. As they do, I move to following them as they carry out their new plan.

"Elevator Ride"

Infrequently, I ask permission of the student to take the lead in a lesson, usually because a strong, persistent idea is in the way of their desire. It is important to note that before making this offer, I will have tried many other ideas. I tell them that I wonder if an "elevator ride" might help create the conditions in which they can conceive of something new for themselves. By elevator ride, I mean that I am choosing, with their permission, to lead and actually move the student toward an unfamiliar option. (If they start to take back the lead, I instantly switch to following.) While I playfully call this an elevator ride, it is not necessarily an up-and-down orientation in movement; it might also be a new angle in limb movement. Immediately after the elevator ride, I ask them to shake it out, then take back the lead of the lesson, thinking and doing the new plan. It is critical that they shake the experience out and use the AT Progression on their own, utilizing the new information. Because each individual coordinates differently, an elevator ride is always an approximation of what is possible. If someone tries to hold on to the elevator ride—either its shape or its feeling—they will get stiff. The function of the elevator ride is as a belief changer, and the learning is complete when the student makes a constructive choice based on the new idea.

New Pathway Maintenance

With an experienced student, I may essentially follow them with my hands for an extended time during an activity—perhaps during a push hands session in tai chi, or while playing a piano concerto, or doing a monologue. They are asking themselves to COORDINATE, and I am using tactile communication to follow their movement process in a flowing learning conversation.

Please Ask

My students report that I have another way I use my hands in teaching. If I think they have stopped thinking amid carrying out their activity, I give them a little one-finger tap to remind them to renew the ask.

One of Many Skills

We teach with our whole selves, and the contribution of skilled tactile communication helps many people learn with their whole selves. We need to ensure that our students do not take on the belief that they need us to use our hands in the teaching process to make a change. The skill of using our hands to teach is valuable to develop and use, and I obviously care deeply about the quality of this aspect of our work. It is one of many skills we use in effective teaching.

Chapter 11

WORD CHOICE

Coincidentally, a studio class I taught the day of this writing high-lighted the powers of word choice, complete with messages that worked and messages gone wrong. We untangled a history of surprising beliefs thanks to the discipline of the AT Progression. When in teaching, you discover many misinterpretations of well-intended messages, the potency of how we deliver our messages becomes crystal clear. Our responsibility to select words with care, to the best of our current knowledge, is reconfirmed.

My Word Choice Principles

My experience is that most of my word choices result from coordinated communication skills—especially listening and omniservation. While I occasionally know the theory supporting the choices I am making as I talk, most of my decisions directly respond to what is happening in the present moment. Following are some of the conscious beliefs, knowledge, and choices that guide my verbal expression. As with many of the teaching skills I have learned, some of these are things "I just did," later finding out from those who watched me what I was doing.

Honesty and Kindness

I was fortunate to study for a time with Cree Elder Eddie Belrose. He spoke of two rules for the Cree People: Honesty and kindness to yourself first, then honestly and kindness to others. As I consider communication of any kind, these are my first guidelines. The questions "What is honest?" and "What is kind?" are frequent visitors to my silent selection process.

Speaking from a "Yes" Perspective

I choose to talk from the "yes"—cooperating with want and desire—whenever possible. On the rare occasion I need to talk from a "don't" perspective, I acknowledge this and elicit my student's help in reframing it as a "yes." Sometimes, the first desire for change comes from something someone doesn't want to do. Until we find a "yes" substitute for what they don't want, however, their coordination will keep reverting to the "don't want" interference. We need to replace the old plan with something more efficacious.

Active versus Passive

Relatively recently, I have begun to question the "let something happen" or "allow something to happen" language sometimes associated with the Alexander Technique. My concern is that such languaging is associated with being a victim, at the mercy of an idea rather than in charge of it. Because we, as Alexander Technique teachers, are advocates of our ability to choose, active voice is more congruent with our principles. Although I don't believe I used much passive language in the past, I now relentlessly choose active phraseology in my teaching. The one more passive phrase I used came from Marj. She would say, in relationship to using your hands to reach for something, "Let the object shape your hands." Because I adopted her wording for so long, saying it in the new way that I have previously described requires conscious attention. What has fascinated me as I omniserve my hands while teaching is that the plan with more active verbs is increasing my skill.

Learning Style Words

I am mildly attentive to a student's choice of words: are they dominantly visual, audio, or kinesthetic? Or even geographic? I say "mildly attentive" because, although I am aware that noticing this gives me clues about how someone prefers to learn, I cannot say that I am deliberately tracking the kind of words I hear. My attention is more individual: "What is this student saying to me now?" And I respond to what I am hearing in that moment. Other people tell me various things I do regarding matching and mismatching preferences. Most of the time, though, my word choices rise simply from being present with the person I am teaching.

I mention *geographic* to note that everyone is unique. I had a student who seemed always to respond in either geographic or cooking terms. Once, when I asked her what she noticed, she replied that her head was in the Arctic and her feet were in Antarctica (clearly demonstrating a Northern Hemisphere bias).

Wholeness

Our work is about the whole self. Unfortunately, our language is not so good at talking whole rather than in parts. One of the first articles I wrote for a professional journal came back several times with my editor asking, "Couldn't we say the mind does this? And the body does that?"—which would have made some of what I was saying simpler. I was steadfast in my reply: "I know that would make the writing prettier, but it would change the meaning—the language needs to reflect wholeness."

When we search for ways to speak whole, we end up with words like *psychophysical* and *biopsychosocial* or even *psychophysicalemotionalspritual*. All sorts of expressions are rife with divisive phrasing such as "I've got to get out of my head" or, conversely, "I've got to get into my body." In my studio, these are delicately banned and reframed. As already mentioned, my occasional use of "minking" and "thoving" is an element of maintaining a whole-self perspective in the room.

Words I "Banish" from the Room

I playfully banish some words from the teaching room. I present a few of these in Table 11.1, with a brief explanation for their banishment. In one class, we actually wrote these words on individual sheets of paper and taped them outside the door of the room. We playfully noted that we left them outside on the way into the studio and were

TEACHING STORY

I am working with a client on preparation for her company's most important yearly fundraising event. She is nervous about standing on stage and speaking in front of several hundred friends, colleagues, and major donors. While we were working, she shared that she'd once been given an instruction by another coach to "not need anything from her audience." Immediately, I had a sense of what behavior that instructor may have hoped to elicit, but then I thought of Cathy's teaching. If this instruction was taken literally, then it suddenly made sense why my client was pulling her body back, away from the audience as she practiced speaking. Using another of Cathy's perspectives on this, I suggested to my client that that particular instruction was a perfect solution for where she was, but now, she's ready for something new. We were able to not make her former instruction "wrong," but rather to celebrate the growth she'd made.

free to pick them up on the way back out if we wanted to. I also occasionally ask someone to "give" me a word, then mime taking it out of the room—again noting that they can have it back later if they want it.

Table 11.1 Banished Words

Banished Words	Brief Explanation
shoulder, waist, hips, neck	These are all anatomically ambiguous terms. We coordinate based on what we are asking ourselves, and, if the ask is for something ambiguous, then our results reflect the lack of clarity.
tension	When people use this word, they tend to sound like some outside force had arrived specially to put pressure or rigidity into them. When they are thinking this way, they become victims. If, instead, they say, "I tighten when I do this…," they realize they are in charge of their choices.
let, allow	See previous discussion on active and passive language. Again, we want to assert agency in our choices.
stress	I describe stress as discoordinating while doing something that you want to do. Generally, when someone says they feel "stressed out" and I ask them what is going on, they are doing things they really want to do, but because "everything is happening at once," they are tightening. It seems to work better to reframe as "I'm choosing to do many things," and to use the Alexander Technique to maximize efficiency in doing them. If they are using stress to say they are having emotional responses, it works better to use the Alexander Technique to coordinate to the emotional response, rather than hurting themselves by tightening.
habit	I banish "habit" sometimes because so many people use the word pejoratively; the truth is that we need habits or we'd have to learn to dress ourselves anew each day.
good, bad, right, wrong	From Marj: "In Alexander's discovery, it isn't a matter of right or wrong, but a matter of observing their habits of sitting" (Stillwell 1981, p.21).
should	"Should" represents a lack of freedom to choose as though imposed by some outside authority.
my head does this and my body does that	"Minking" and "thoving" is the replacement for this. Every action is a whole-self event. A dance that celebrates wholeness can be used in class anytime someone says anything that is self-divisive.

open/closed	This frequently comes up when someone blames their arms for something "postural": they start pulling their arms back to be "open" rather than "closed." I have taken to being a bit graphic about this one: "If you succeed in opening, you will be bloody." We need to redefine what they actually mean by "open" and how that physiologically manifests in a coordinated way.
inside/outside	Similarly, we can't go "inside." Nor do we want to examine our liver. What do we really mean?
vulnerable	This is a scary word for most people. It makes us think we are "bait" for someone to hurt. Understanding the beneficent intention when people use it, I think that what it really means is "able and willing to respond to stimuli." That sounds much more appealing to me.
pubic bone and sitz bone	Perhaps this is more a caution rather than a fully banned word. A student recently realized from a question I asked her that she thought the "public bone" and "sitz bone" were separate from the pelvis. The way they are named does makes it sound like they are separate bones, rather than names for parts of the bone. Sitz bone is also problematic because: (1) many people mistake it for their hip joint and try to move from a nonmoving part; (2) some people try to balance over their ischial tuberosity (the replacement word for sitz bone) rather than over the hip joint.
stage fright	I fervently wish that these two words had never been put together. The increased needs of performance can create an energized state that, because it is similar to a fright reaction, is often misinterpreted. We need a highly energized state to do extraordinary things. Chapter 6 in my book for performers discusses this in depth (Madden 2014). Recently, I have coined a new word—sidere—to acknowledge this liminal state (see Chapter 30).
breathing low	Many people limit their breathing by trying—impossibly—to force air into their abdomen while keeping their ribs rigid. They are surprised, and sometimes shocked, when I point out that the lungs are entirely inside the ribs. Breathe whole, breathe whole, breathe whole!
grounded	We are always grounded because gravity works, simple as that. When someone is told that they need to be "grounded" it is generally because they are tightening in a way that has thrown them off balance, making their feet and legs work extra hard to keep them from falling. Restoring coordination restores cooperation with gravity.

Invented Words

Throughout this book, you've been introduced to words I have invented. In my teaching studio, the central invented word is an active verb that we devise to invite ourselves to cooperate with our design. This is the word that represents the initiation of the AT Progression, for which I have used in this book COORDINATE in small caps. After years of varieties of experiments with language, I find my students are most successful (in the speed of understanding) if the chosen word is new and thus unattached to preconceived meanings. It seems beneficial that the word also be playful. The first time I used a made-up word in a beginners class, I was astounded by how fast they learned. Having no meaning associated with the chosen verb enables the students to think creatively, with no idea of attaining a particular end result or feeling.

Some of the invented verbs I have used in my teaching are found in the first chapter; here are others: soleil, anosea, pepla, ctenophore, momo, kirribilli, m'walla, danjillie, and many more. Personally, I find having many verbs for this process has built up my own skills and flexibility. Inventing a shared word in a group setting involves everyone in the decision, which is a key element in successful adult learning groups. (This is discussed further in Chapter 22.)

Reframing

In the video about Marj broadcast by Nebraska Educational Television, there is a moment while playing the violin when the student (Cynthia Mauney) looks surprised and says, "That's very different…" Marj replies, "It's different, but it's fun" (Barstow 2009). While saying "yes" to the student's perception, she also renames it as fun rather than different. I often reframe while teaching. Sometimes, my students might not directly notice it; other times, they realize and know why I am doing it. Eventually, they start to reframe for themselves:

> To understand why it's there, it helps to perceive a problem in a new way; get a different slant on it, see it in a new light, put another spin on it… *Reframing* is a way of changing your perception of an experience—changing the meaning by changing the way it is presented. (Linden and Perutz 2008, p.207)

Sometimes, a reframe is as simple as replacing one of the aforenamed banished words. For example, if someone says their shoulder movement is restricted, I might say, "Let's see how your arm moves as you do that motion." Or, I may point to a new concept altogether: if I ask a performer what she does before going onstage and she says "relax," I might offer instead, "What you really want is a coordinated state of excitement—readiness."

Our Words Are Windows to Our Beliefs

Omniserving what someone says with what is happening in the head–spine relationship while they say it often yields an important clue or a cue to ask a question. If a word they are using is useful for learning, it stays in the room; if it corresponds with interference, it is kindly escorted out.

As students deepen in understanding the Alexander Technique, some invent their own words for body parts or concepts—they have experienced that renaming things aids in thinking them anew. It is not uncommon in a class for someone to start to say something, realize that it is somehow not helping them, and look for new ways. Or, to start a turn, realize that the words they are thinking are causing them to discoordinate, and sit back down—they have learned what they needed to learn. When this happens, my job becomes simply to be with them as they teach themselves.

Chapter 12

THE ART OF THE QUESTION

Remember that you are always the one who knows the least about what is happening with your student. Your students have the answers—your job is to ask the questions.

Questions and Whole-Self Listening

In the Living Room Étude, Marj's offer as I finished each teaching lesson was, "Why don't you think about that for a while?" Her question was asking me to ask myself questions. Eventually, I learned the art of self-curiosity, which I might describe as nonjudgmental questioning of myself. My ability to approach self-inquiry with as much honesty and kindness as I could muster gave me the initial skills I needed to formulate questions for my students.

Beyond the social hellos, I almost always begin workshops, classes, and lessons with questions. To create the conditions in which I know that I am teaching what my student wants to learn requires that I get some information from them:

What are you interested in today?

What brought you here today?

How can I help you?

What questions are you bringing with you today?

What have you been working on lately?

What might the next step in your journey be?

Beginning with questions emphasizes that in my learning playground, the desire that drives the learning belongs to the students. I want to communicate clearly that they are perfect as they are, and while I am ready and willing to assist them, any desire to learn, experiment, or make any changes originates with their desire. These opening queries also promote an atmosphere of curiosity in the room.

In introductory classes, I warn students, "I ask a lot of questions. You can answer in any way—including 'I don't know' or 'I won't tell you.' I ask the questions to seek information that might help in the lesson, or if I need clarification." Choosing whether to respond to my potential barrage of questions gives students another way to exercise the connection of coordination with freedom to choose.

Listening—in the sense of whole-self-reception—is at the heart of the art of the question. As I ask myself to use the Alexander Technique to invite my students to be with me while I am with them so that I can omniserve what is happening (looking, listening, possibly moving with) so that I can wonder what would create the environment in which they can learn what they want to learn, I am looking for clues.

My first task is to receive the information. Actors are trained in this. In a BBC interview, Alan Rickman says that his mantra to young actors is, "You only speak because you wish to respond to something you have heard," and adds, "I want to see the intensity and accuracy of their listening." He, like me, conceives of listening as a whole-self event. He asks, "How alive are you to your fellow actors?" (Rickman 2010). The whole-self-reception skills I learned as an actor/director were potentized as I started to use the Alexander Technique to listen; the omniservation skills I learned so as to teach the Alexander Technique potentized my whole-self-reception skills as an actor/director. Win-win.

TEACHING STORY
During one lesson at the Friday Harbor workshop, I was wanting to tell a story, and having a bit of a clunky time getting going. Cathy was standing next to me and reminded me, "You know this," offering me an unspoken question. The release I experienced in getting that "Yes!" moment and how it unfolded was wonderful.

Store Clerks (Again) and Others

I practice listening when in the day-to-day interactions of shopping or traveling. At the time of this writing, I am out of town and just dined in a restaurant with a common table. I got to experience the story of someone tracing his family history back several centuries; apparently, the woman he was talking to was a relative he was meeting for the first time. Discreetly noticing their interchange, I omniserved a dance of excitement and common bonds affecting coordination and movement.

Responding to what words you actually hear in these daily moments offers an opportunity for playful practice. In acting training, many exercises ask you to verbally name or describe what you are receiving/experiencing. Whole-self-listening is another skill that began in my acting training and now serves my teaching. A simple solo game (which can also be done with a partner) is to listen to a story (live or recorded) and say, in as close a time as possible, the exact words you are hearing.

Listening Filters for Teaching

Several well-practiced filters help me organize the information I receive. The most primary has been covered in this book from a variety of angles: What are they actually doing and saying? How are they moving as they speak? Does their coordination significantly shift at any point in what they are saying?

> *Although I have said this many times already, I can't stress it enough: your students will always know more about what is going on than you do. If you try to analyze the information before you fully receive it, you aren't getting the information you need.*

As I am listening, I utilize two filters concurrently to informally organize the information I receive. The first group of questions regards the circumstance of the lesson and student, while the second sorts what we are hearing for viability as a successful change plan or action plan. I don't necessarily expect to receive answers to all the questions, yet I am prepared to hear any of the answers I need, wondering if they will be useful in the lesson. If a question is unanswered but seems to be pertinent, the fact that its answer is missing might be the clue I need and lead to a question I might ask the student. In Table 12.1, the filters are charted side by side to highlight their simultaneity.

Table 12.1 Listening Filters

Circumstance Questions (adapted from actor training for teaching, see particularly Uta Hagen) (Hagen 1973)	Change Plan Questions (adapted from NLP/Linden) (Linden and Perutz 2008)
Who are we?	Is it constructive?
Who are we with (if applicable)?	Is it possible?
If it is a group, what group am I with?	Is it within the student's control?
Where am I teaching? Where does the situation the student is describing take place?	Is it ecological? (a) Is it healthy for the student? (Or does it hurt them?)
What time is it? What time does the situation the student is describing take place?	Is it ecological? (b) Is it healthy for others? (Or does it hurt anyone else?)
What people and objects are in your current environment? What people and objects are in the situation the student is describing?	Is it ecological? (c) Is it respectful of the environment, the world? (Or does it hurt anything?)
What is the likely sequence of events in the situation your student is describing?	
What does your student want for the lesson?	
How does the lesson relate to the students' longer-range goals/life goals?	
What does the student perceive is in the way?	
What actions has the student taken already?	

This may seem like a lot to sort through. In truth, it is just bringing to consciousness information you are already receiving. As an actor, I often practiced answering the Circumstance Questions for different characters in plays and people in daily life, sometimes focusing on only one of the questions. If this type of listening–listening in order to receive and sort the information consciously–is new to you, then one way to begin playing with it might be to ask these questions about a character in a story or novel. You could also practice by picking one of the questions to wonder about as you go about your daily life. The filters analyze the information we are already receiving so that pertinent elements are available for constructive planning in the teaching playground. Practice creates facility.

Notes about the Change Plan Questions

When I first started teaching people to teach the Alexander Technique, I realized there were some things I just "knew" were a good idea but didn't know how to explain why. For a short while, I asked a trusted colleague who knew Neuro-Linguistic Programming (NLP) to watch me teach and offer ideas about how to explain my process. While I never formally studied it, the information my colleague gave me helped me explain some of what I do in teaching. For example, he saw me create plans for change that matched the NLP criteria for change plans:

1. Constructive, with constructive being identified as pursuing what you want (rather than avoiding what you don't want). In my current words, this would be a "yes" plan.

2. Possible, meaning that you can accomplish it. (For instance, I could help an expert skier create a plan to ski moguls that would be possible for them. If I gave myself the same plan, it would be an impossible one at my current level of skiing skills.)

3. Within your control, meaning that you are in charge of the outcome. This is of key importance for teachers. Whether somebody learns is out of our control; we can only create the best invitation to learning that we can come up with.

4. Ecological, referring to the fact that it doesn't hurt you, anyone else, or anything. In reviewing Linden's work, I ascertain that this question really addresses how your change fits into your biopsychosocial world. "By ecological I mean our personal ecology, the interrelating systems we are composed of... In estimating the future impact of your outcome, you have to consider, in addition to the advantages you expect, the possible disadvantages that even the most desired and well-formed outcome may bring" (Linden and Perutz 2008, p.121). I framed *ecological* in two ways in the preceding chart—healthy versus hurtful. It is a more pointed version of the question on the circumstance side of the chart—"How does the lesson

relate to the students' longer-range goals/life goals?" because you are also doing a values analysis. Not only "What do I want?" but also "How does what I want serve my greater world?" (For further discussion, see Chapters 18–26 in Linden and Perutz 2008.)

Once I knew these change plan criteria, it was fascinating to discover that any time someone tried to do an activity that didn't meet these standards, they tightened between head and spine. These criteria have become measures for considering whether someone's plan for themselves is healthy and sustainable.

Another Possible Filter

If the student is doing the activity while talking about what they want, then I also am listening/omniserving with the Analysis of Activity tools of Chapter 9. What exactly are they doing? In what sequence are they doing it? How would I describe their coordination while they do it? What is happening between head and spine? What is making how it is happening perfect? What do I know, if anything, about the activity, skill, or question they have? Have I done it myself? Have I taught anyone else who does this or something like it? What do I know about human design that might contribute to this request? Do I know any resources that might be helpful? Are they available?

I learned to use these guiding filters gradually, selecting particular questions to focus on while adding them one by one to my tool kit. In the integrative whole-self creativity I talk about in Part Three, the questions "dance" as I omniserve; the filters help me select what might prove important to pursue.

With my first analysis tools, all questions, my curiosity and wonder are awake. I am reminded of Rainer Maria Rilke's thoughts on questions:

> have patience with everything unresolved in your heart and try to love the questions themselves as if they were locked rooms or books written in a foreign language. Don't search for the answers, which could not be given to you now, because you would not be able to live them. And the point is to live everything. *Live* the questions now. Perhaps then, someday far in the future, you will gradually,

without even noticing it, live your way into the answer. (Rilke 1986, pp.34–35; original emphasis)

Watching one of my theatre mentors, Richard Nichols, teaching a class, I suddenly had an "aha!" moment about asking questions. I was watching him search for a means to coach someone, and realized, "He's asking questions because he doesn't know the answers!" Prior to that moment, I essentially attributed omniscience to excellent teachers. Realizing that what was contributing to Richard's expertise was innocence of the answers freed me to become a naïve, curious questioner.

Chapter 13

STORYTELLING

Stories arise from the world of play. We get to know each other more through exchanging narratives of our days. We entertain each other with stories. And from the time we were children, we have learned through story. In teaching, stories could be called the "citations" of the spoken word—they provide the reference that shores up proffered new paradigms.

An Alexander Technique teaching story has...

1. A beginning, with a problem to solve.

2. A middle, the narrative of how the problem was addressed.

3. An end, with either a successful resolution of the problem or a successful redefinition of the problem that will lead to eventual success.

The story's intent is honest and kind. It contains specific circumstances, sensory content, and sometimes humor, perhaps illustrating specific Alexander Technique or other learning principles.

F.M. Alexander gave us a beautiful example of a teaching story: His chapter "Evolution of a Technique" tells of his discovery of the work. His story includes all of the aforementioned elements. For each of us, our own rendition of his story is a potent teaching tool.

Your own version of how you came to study the Alexander Technique and what it has done for you is one you will share over and over again. If you tell it as a teaching story, consider consciously constructing it to include all of the previous elements. My own Alexander Technique story has several versions, including one that is theatre-based and one that is teaching-based. I can use the theatre story to relate to any profession by selecting elements from it that match the wants, needs, and desires of my participants. I have reworked, rehearsed, and honed both these stories to tell the story I want to tell. Because we have lived the biopsychosocial history of our Alexander Technique journey, we cellularly relate to what we are saying, inviting our audience to live the story with us as we tell it.

Some of my stories reappear many times; they are well rehearsed and their content has been carefully selected over time. Other stories may have only one appearance in my teaching studio. Many of the stories are directly related to events in my life, while some are learned from someone or somewhere else.

Rehearsed Stories

Like F.M. Alexander's meticulously crafted story, and my own story of coming to the Alexander Technique, I have a set of teaching stories that I have developed and rehearsed. While they vary somewhat with each group, their elements have been crafted specifically to meet common Alexander Technique questions. When telling these stories, I tell them as though it was the first time (which is much easier to do if you have actually rehearsed them).

Here is one of those stories—Ron's story (I have attached his first name to it with his permission). When searching for a new way to do my introduction to the Alexander Technique, I remembered this event and realized that it would illustrate the work well to beginners. *I annotate the story with my rationale in italics.*

Ron's Story

This story appears in an introduction after I have made the often-surprising assertion, "At the outset of a change process, it is important to know that we do perfectly what we do based on the information we have."

An actor at the university helped me to understand this in a deep way.

I identify myself as a teacher willing to learn from her students, which supports building relationship with adult learners.

He was having a great deal of trouble with his voice, and the faculty was not going to cast him in a play, which is unusual in our program.

The problem.

It was obvious that he was tightening significantly in the relationship between head and spine, and the other faculty members asked me about this. My response was, "I know, but he hates the Alexander Technique."

That I am talking about someone "hating" the Alexander Technique reassures people that I am fine with however they respond to the work. It reinforces freedom to choose. It also puts me in the "problem" because I have colleagues who want Ron to learn something new.

He did seem to hate class, and would sit scowling in the darkest corner of the studio.

Usually, as I tell this, I imitate him, adding a little humor and movement to the moment. Sensory content vivifies the story. If I am telling this story at the university, I also mention the room number, because it is a really dark room, with corners one could hide in.

The next class, I said to him, "You know that we are concerned about your voice, and I know you don't like the Alexander Technique. But I think it could help. Can we have another experiment?' He grunted an "okay."

This interchange sets up a classroom where the student is in charge, in the lead. My new group hears me asking for permission to offer new information. I am now in the second phase of the teaching story–the process towards a solution.

This time, as he used the Alexander Technique, he changed just a little, and he turned and looked at me and said, "My Mom always said I would lose my head if I didn't keep it on." In that moment, he looked about 5 years old, even though he was 25.

Again, I imitate the movement of his look at me–usually some people gasp or laugh as they recognize the situation.

We realized that what he was doing was perfect for a five-year-old who thought he was going to lose his head. Previously, he had no recollection why he was tightening between head and spine. He just knew it was frightening not to do it.

As he realized what he had been thinking, he was alternately frightened and amused. I reassured him that his head would stay on, and, laughing, he agreed, then was immediately able to coordinate between head and spine. Discovering this information provided the next step in the solution to the problem.

He had a great time that week with his updated information: his voice improved almost immediately, and he spent a good deal of time laughing because he had to keep reminding himself that his head would stay on.

Using the Alexander Technique solved the problem, and the result was successful and enjoyable. While the story began with what might be called troublesome moments in teaching and learning, the journey through the difficulty was well worth it.

With his previous information, tightening between head and spine was perfect; with his new information, a flexible relationship between head and spine was perfect.

With this I am emphasizing the reason I told the story, again assuring the learning cohort that I believe everyone in the room is perfect.

Ron's story has all of the elements I mentioned earlier: he had a problem that he decided to address with the Alexander Technique process I offered; the process revealed more information, which reinforced his ability to use the Alexander Technique successfully to address the problem. My relationship to the student in the story—Ron—demonstrates the honesty and kindness that guides my classroom choices. It has sensory and movement details, while including a bit of humor. The perfect-to-perfect arc of the story affirms compassion in the learning community while teaching a necessary understanding of how humans learn.

Storytelling researcher Jonas Sach notes that, "human beings share stories to remind each other of who they are and how they should act" (p.4), and that, "So many of the stories that have really stuck, that have shaped culture, are about one thing: people reaching for their highest potential and struggling to create a better world" (p.8). Every Alexander Technique class embodies the reach for that highest potential. The simple formula that Sach offers is "derived from the wisdom storytellers have employed since the beginning of time... preserved in the 'three commandments' laid out in 1895 by marketing's first great storyteller, John Powers: *Tell the Truth, Be Interesting, and Live the Truth*" (Sachs 2012, p.8; original emphasis).

These simple guidelines are an excellent match to teaching the Alexander Technique, because in using the Alexander Technique to teach the Alexander Technique, we are "living our truth."

One of the components mentioned may not be immediately clear: How do specific circumstances and sensory content help in creating teaching stories? From Powers's formulation, they relate to the "be interesting" part. I illustrate this, contrasting two descriptions of what I am doing right now:

One: I am sitting at my desk typing on my computer.

Two: My cat is purring in his basket on the edge of my desk, a refinished table from my graduate school days. Windows on two sides display the vivid green of evergreen trees against the background of Seattle's gray winter sky. A zinging alert about someone's birthday coincidentally appeared on my laptop while I was writing about the importance of sensory detail in story.

Both are true. I would guess that as you read the second account, you created your own picture of where I am, possibly reacting to sensory elements that appeal or don't appeal to you. The sensory detail invites you to be participatory in the story.

Such specific detail in stories encourages active engagement, often eliciting an emotional response—all of which aids retention and enjoyment. Storytelling has been a part of human culture as far back as we can track. Evolutionary psychologist Jonathan Gottschall says:

Until recently we've only been able to speculate about story's persuasive effects. But over the last several decades psychology has begun a serious study of how story affects the human mind. Results repeatedly show that our attitudes, fears, hopes, and values are strongly influenced by story. (Gottschall 2012)

How Do Stories Assist in Teaching the Alexander Technique?

Content aside, telling a story creates a communication bridge between teacher and students, and between students and teachers. We want our students to feel free to tell their stories so that we have the information we need to help them learn what they want to learn. One way to create such an environment is to model it: if I tell a story, then stories are welcome!

I use stories simply to help get people talking to each other, to back up facts with a vivid description of a successful use of that information, to offer a parallel story, or to help someone who is struggling with a new idea. I use them to let people know I have done some research or learned from someone else, too. I use them to recount the successful use of new ideas. I use them to change the pace or mood, if needed. Some of my stories are fairly long and have been carefully constructed, like Ron's story. Others last only one sentence.

I have learned to tell a story most of the time when I happen to think of it while teaching. Every so often, I say, "I don't know why I want to tell this story, but I keep thinking of it." It still surprises me how often I find out that the story matches someone's question or need.

Balance is important. As with all teaching processes, the art of using stories effectively evolves through analysis and practice. For the students who prefer to learn by watching and listening, stories are especially important. For the folks who want to move, you want to make sure your stories contain a lot of vivid detail and that you balance talking and doing.

Here are a few more of my stories, charted to illustrate the elements mentioned at the head of the chapter (Tables 13.1–13.3).

The story in Table 13.1 invites people to include more possibilities for change when they use the Alexander Technique.

Table 13.1 Story Chart 1

Elements	Story
A beginning with a problem to solve	A scene designer keeps running in and out of the theater in which I am teaching an introduction to the Alexander Technique. What I don't find out until later is that he was trying to solve a design problem—and was paying attention to what I was saying.
A story of how the problem was addressed	As the actors were leaving, he came up to me and asked if I would give him a lesson while he was looking at the stage.
A successful resolution of the process	As he used the Alexander Technique, his eyes lit up, then he ran quickly to his design table, exclaiming, "Now I can see it!"
Honesty and kindness	A core value in my teaching, possibly exemplified here by my choosing to stay and teach him as well.

Specific circumstances, sensory content, humor	He is running in and out of the room. The words "theater," "stage," and "design table" evoke a sense of place.
Specific Alexander Technique examples	Whole self, application to vision, creative process.

The story in Table 13.2 explains how studied rehearsed plans intended for one activity may get in the way in other activities, in this case causing discomfort. This might also be a good story when the class includes a couple.

Table 13.2 Story Chart 2

Elements	Story
A beginning with a problem to solve	A woman had been coming for lessons for some time, and one of our puzzles was some consistent, persistent pattern in her arm movement. One day, her husband came with her and sat quietly in the corner of the room, reading.
A story of how the problem was addressed	As his wife and I were exploring different patterns of arm movement, the man suddenly burst out laughing. She and I looked at him quizzically. He looked at me and said, "She used to be a weaver. She keeps her arms like that all the time, and I just realized they are exactly as they need to be to move the shuttle back and forth. She even carries the laundry basket that way."
A successful resolution of the process	His omniservation was exactly what his wife and I needed. She used the Alexander Technique to imaginatively "put the shuttle down." Immediately, many more arm movements were available to her.
Honesty and kindness	Everyone in the room was honest and kind.
Specific circumstances, sensory content, humor	The couple in the room, the husband sitting in the corner of the room reading, the weaving, the shuttle, the laundry basket, the laughter.
Specific Alexander Technique examples	Illustrates biopsychosocial history's role in how we coordinate ourselves, while highlighting that a little detective work might be needed to discover the new constructive plan.

The story in Table 13.3 offers the possibility of trusting the process rather than looking for an end result.

Table 13.3 Story Chart 3

Elements	Story
A beginning with a problem to solve	Marj had come to Seattle to do a workshop. Most of the people in the room were friends who had studied with her over a number of years. At the first coffee break, everyone was visiting—laughing, talking loudly—and it really was quite raucous in the room. Marj looked at me and told me it was time to gather everyone to start again, then kept watching me. This created a little performance anxiety for me because she was watching to see how I would handle the situation.
A story of how the problem was addressed	I created my plan and carried it through: using the Alexander Technique to pitch my voice a little higher than usual (knowing that would help acoustically) as I invited everyone in the room to be with me as I moved air to call, "Time to come back!" My first thought after the words were out of my mouth was, "Uh-oh"—I didn't feel I had done enough for everyone to hear me.
A successful resolution of the process	Everyone stopped talking, immediately. Despite feeling I hadn't succeeded, I obviously had succeeded.
Honesty and kindness	I had to choose to be honest and kind to myself to carry out my plan while Marj was watching me.
Specific circumstances, sensory content, humor	The room, the excitement, the coffee, Marj's gaze, the pitch of my voice.
Specific Alexander Technique examples	An immediate need to reason out a means-whereby and follow it through, step by step, without "checking in" to see if it is working.

As I teach, I receive the gift of more and more stories.

Chapter 14

CHOICE

Implicit at every step of teaching the Alexander Technique is embodying the confidence that choice is available and possible for everyone. My hope is that people rediscover freedom from patterns they think they're stuck with or "are just them." We can inadvertently end up with such limiting beliefs. Sometimes, new students need to "grow" into knowing choice is possible. While they might need some time to become fluent with the Alexander Technique process, they always know it is possible to figure out a constructive plan. When teachers hold the belief that choice is possible for everyone in the room, the experience of choice is available to all participants.

When I was teaching a workshop in Alaska, a woman arrived late and was semi-pushed into the room by her daughter. She was angry! It seems she had been virtually kidnapped from her kitchen while busy making a meal for an event. Her daughter had taken my introduction the day before and "knew" that the Alexander Technique was what her mother needed.

I kept teaching for a while, silently inviting her into the group, including her in all the communication. She was one of the most "tight"-looking people I had ever seen. Everything seemed rigidly held in place. After she had had some time to experience the freedom of choice in the room, I asked her why she thought her daughter had been so adamant. She gave a litany of the many injuries she had had in recent years—mostly broken bones of many varieties—and, I thought, "Ah, I see why it is perfect (though not actually helpful) for her to hold herself in place. She has experienced a lot of things 'falling apart.'" I reviewed the introductory information about the Alexander Technique (as she had missed it), and asked if she wanted a turn. She agreed. Her first words after her first experiment were, "Oh, I didn't know I was tight!" I was amazed; although she was experiencing pain in her daily life, she literally didn't know she was tight. To her credit (with a nod to her daughter's brash wisdom), she cancelled everything she could cancel that weekend in order to attend the rest of the workshop, and enjoyed the freedom to make new choices.

Prior to the workshop, she didn't know anything else was possible; choice had disappeared. A key moment was when, after supplying some information, I gave her a choice about having a turn. If she said "no," then I would thank her and tell her she was welcome to stay or go. By asking her first, I was modeling freedom to choose.

I need a clear "yes, I want to learn" before I offer a lesson. The first thing we teach—that we have a choice—is important; we can teach nothing else if the students don't believe they have a choice. *Skilled integrated choice* might be another three-word description of the Alexander Technique.

For our students to experience freedom, they must know that we, as teachers, are okay if they choose not to learn what we want to teach. Years ago, someone asked one of my students what she thought my underlying message as a teacher was. She said, "Cathy's message is 'You can if you want to, but you don't have to.'" What she said resonated with me. That phrase conveys belief in the student, a request for desire, and freedom to choose. "You don't have to" carried the implication "Cathy will be fine with that, too." And I must be. If I am not, I am not offering my students the same freedom of choice that I cherish for myself.

A great deal of neuroscience research is in progress on the nature of mind and consciousness and many questions about the nature of choice and will. In reviewing it, I note that even when the researchers question the nature of free will, they don't suggest we abandon it. Daniel Siegel says, "A marvelous reality we seem to have encountered is that we are not passive in all this activity of mind and awareness. With consciousness comes the possibility of choice and change" (Siegel 2017, p.266). Jon Lieff, a practicing neuropsychiatrist and specialist in the interface of psychiatry, neurology, and medicine, noted in an online review of *The Volitional Brain*:

> Benjamin Libet contributed to the notion that there is no free will by finding that 200 milliseconds before we act the unconscious brain displays a signal of the future action. He is the editor of this volume of essays where he tries to set the record straight about his view that

although the unconscious may start the process, there is still a conscious veto power that does leave open the notion of free will. (Lieff n.d.)

When people query me about free will or say there is no free will, they often refer to Libet's study. However, Libet says:

> My conclusion about free will, one genuinely free in the non-determined sense, is then that its existence is at least as good, if not a better, scientific option than its denial by determinist theory. Given the speculative nature of both determinist and non-determinist theories, why not adopt the view that we do have free will (until some real contradictory evidence may appear, if it ever does). Such a view would at least allow us to proceed in a way that accepts and accommodates our own deep feeling that we do have a free will. (Libet 2004, p.56)

TEACHING STORY

Unexpectedly, I had an opportunity to audition for a professional theatre company I'd wanted to work with for years. Despite the ease in scheduling and arranging brush-up coaching sessions, something was off. I could not wholly get behind my own decision to do the audition. It wasn't fear of the outcome, it was fear that this had become an outdated ask for something I no longer wanted. But, because I wasn't able to fully admit this, I dutifully practiced. And, as a result, I seemed to be transported several years back to habits I was certain I'd already eradicated. My mind could justify all the perfect reasons for me to commit to this decision, but my body was not believing any of it. I did not seem able to come into coordination around this. Cathy reminded me of the freedom of choice. The only decision I needed to make each time I went to practice, was that I desired to do this work now, today, not for the rest of my life. And it was this freedom that helped me recognize that this potential job was not an active desire. I cancelled. There were no consequences, and I was able to focus my attention in a different direction.

All of which is to say that the researcher many people reference when they dispute free will does not draw that conclusion himself. In the time before I could counter Libet with Libet, I would respond that whatever the answer regarding free will, if we practiced using the Alexander Technique consistently, whatever happens in that "200 milliseconds before we act" would improve in coordination.

It is so important that the student be willful in this process because the heart of our work requires a conscious choice to say "yes" to a new idea—the willful "yes." If we say "yes" to our new plan, the previous plan has disappeared. Sometimes, I explain this to a group by saying, "If I am walking to the door, and I want to do something different, then I either walk to the desk, or decide to stand, or perhaps dance. The only way I stop walking to the door is to do something else—to say 'yes' to something else."

The same is true in our thought processes. How do you stop thinking something? You think of something else. A colleague, Ken Anno, made me a wonderful pipe cleaner creation of a turquoise spotted platypus to illustrate a point I continually make: "If you don't want to think of a pink elephant, you need to think of something else, perhaps a turquoise spotted platypus."

If a student arrives and wants me to decide what activity to do, I won't. I might offer, "Would you like to do this or that?" to help narrow the choices, but I am still asking for a willful "yes." Occasionally, someone really doesn't want to choose; then, I—honestly, kindly—say we have nothing to do, and if it is a group class move on to someone else. These rare occasions become the lesson. In part, the student may be acting out of a pedagogical model in which they expect the teacher to tell them what to do. Or they may be thinking in a medical model in which the health care practitioner tells them what to do. In either case, my declining to make their choice for them is the first step in teaching the Alexander Technique, the first essential exercise of the freedom to choose. And, often, the desire does emerge once the student really knows they have the choice.

Many of the games in "Games Digest" involve choices. I particularly use the maze games to play with coordinating at the moment of choice. A simple game to introduce choice in a class is to ask everyone to stand behind their chair (assuming the chairs are in a circle). Their next task is to walk to the center of the circle. Before they do that, ask each one to plan: Are they going to the right or the left of the chair? Remind them that they could choose to stay where they are. In the first round of this game, simply say "go" and everyone can carry out their actions. For the second round, ask everyone to select an option again—it can be the same or a different plan. This time, when you say "go," everyone can do what they planned or switch in the moment to one of the other choices. Most groups will spontaneously start to discuss what they noticed when they renewed freedom of choice. You can play this quite a few times because people enjoy playing with the variations. For a bit more fun, you can put simple toys or chocolates in the middle for players to collect when they get there.

Lieff, the neuropsychiatrist I referred to earlier, offers that, "Conscious free will does exist, but must be found and exercised. It is like training a new muscle" (Lieff 2013).

This could be yet another three-word definition of Alexander Technique: a free-will exerciser.

Chapter 15

WHOLENESS IN THE BIOPSYCHOSOCIAL WAY

I was recently introduced to a term used in medicine—*biopsychosocial*—introduced by physician George Engel, Professor of Medicine and Psychiatry at the University of Rochester Medical Center. From Engel:

> I have proposed guidelines for a more inclusive model, a biopsychosocial model based on general systems theory. As the name suggests, its intent is to provide a framework within which can be conceptualized and related as natural systems all the levels of organization pertinent to health and disease, from subatomic particles through molecules, cells, tissues, organs, organ systems, the person, the family, the community, the culture and ultimately, the biosphere.
>
> …Overall health reflects a high level of intra- and intersystemic harmony. Such harmony may be disrupted at any level, at the cellular, at the organ system, at the whole person or at the community levels. Whether the resulting disturbance is contained at the level at which it is initiated or whether other levels become implicated is a function of the capacity of that system to adjust to change. (Engel 1978, p.175)

To me, this term encompasses what I experience as I teach the Alexander Technique more completely than Alexander's term *psychophysical*. His own story in "The Evolution of a Technique" has *bio* (his voice), *psycho* (his anger, his despair, his consternation, his determination, his intellect), and *social* (theatre, the doctor, his father, his voice teacher) elements. When I teach, all of these factors are woven into the lessons.

While the word is quite new to me in my teaching, I have found enough success saying "biopsychosocial" in the last few months that it is gradually replacing *psychophysical* in my teaching vocabulary.

The term also encompasses the kinds of stories that emerge, often unexpectedly, in Alexander Technique lessons. Lynne Compton's story about a lesson about arm movement is an example:

> Cathy suggested that her teachers-in-training collect a few stories to illustrate different teaching ideas. This story surfaced during my training, and I sometimes share it with students. In a class we were playing with noticing our movement as we rolled a large air-filled exercise ball around the room. Cathy noticed some extra work as I reached out and suggested some changes in my coordination. As my movement became easier, a memory of a doll I had played with as a young child flashed into my consciousness. In the 1950s, some dolls were constructed from a hard material and the legs, arms, and head were attached to the torso by a system of elastic bands. In the interior of the doll's torso area, a hook was incorporated in the design. Similar hooks were molded into each limb and the interior of the head. Thick rubber bands stretched from the hook in the torso into each limb and the head. Turning the doll's head or having her sit or reach for something would eventually lead to the rubber bands weakening and snapping. Then her legs, arms, or head would fall off, and my parents would have to perform surgery with a crochet hook to replace the snapped rubber bands. These operations had varying degrees of success.
>
> In the class as I reached out towards the rolling ball with an easier coordination, I understood that my earlier movement had been colored by the thought that I had better keep my arm well attached or an interior elastic band might snap and my arm would fall off!

Her arm movement had been affected by a fear of her arm falling off, based on the kind of doll she had: *bio*—her movement choices; *psycho*—her fear; *social*—the doll in her childhood home.

Another example comes from a time I used my hands to invite an actor to some more free arm movement. He suddenly changed and I knew something significant had shifted. Based on the look in his eyes, I asked him, "Where are we?" He told me we were underwater. I asked him what was happening and he said, "There is a shark." I had touched him exactly where his friend had touched him when they were scuba diving and saw a shark, and he had suddenly been transported back to that frightening event. I talked him back to land, took care of the fear by asking him to see where he really was, and continued exploring arm movement back in a safe environment. Biopsychosocial again.

In an extended story in *Direction* magazine, naturopathic doctor Mary Gallagher described using the Alexander Technique to create new neural pathways to respond to recurring episodes of Post-Traumatic Stress Disorder. This is a detailed look at all three elements of *biopsychosocial*. She began her discovery in an acting class I was co-teaching:

> As part of an exercise, we were extending our arms repeatedly. The movement stimulated memories of past abuse. The Alexander teacher came over to me. She asked me to ask my neck "to take a vacation" so that my head would not be pressing down on my spine. Next she worked with my arms and body to help me find a new way to reach out. This time it didn't stimulate the old memory. Eureka! I had found a way to construct new neural pathways. (Gallagher 2005, p.27)

In none of the above lessons was I seeking a deeper meaning. I was just helping with arm movement. (It is coincidental that I picked three stories involving arms.) With the latter story, I didn't know until much later what had transpired for her in that lesson.

(Interestingly, in Gallagher's story, you can see that I was using different words for teaching at the time. Another definition of the Alexander Technique might be "personal evolution tool.")

The neural pathways of our lives are literally etched in our selves. Daniel Coyle's examination of deep practice includes a discussion of how we create new skilled pathways in a process called "myelination." He notes that once a pathway had been forged, "Myelin wraps—it doesn't unwrap. Like a highway paving machine, myelination happens in one direction. Once a skill is insulated, you can't un-insulate it (except through age or disease)... The only way to change them is to build new habits by repeating new behaviors—by myelinating new circuits" (Coyle 2009, pp.44–45).

> **TEACHING STORY**
> In a private lesson, Cathy helped me to process a childhood trauma. While I verbally relived the experience with intense fright and anger, her gentle hands kept reminding me that I am no longer a vulnerable little child, but a capable adult. That lesson allowed me to embody what I had learned in years of therapy, and enabled me to heal that childhood trauma.

While myelination is just one aspect of creating neural pathways, the structure of the AT Progression in a lesson does just what Coyle suggests: we choose and practice new skilled behaviors, changing our biopsychosocial responses.

All lessons are biopsychosocial. Some, as those above, carry a bit more resonance in a person's life. The AT Progression remains the organizing structure for what I think of as walking with the person at the moment of a significant revelation. Usually, the pace of the lesson either slows down or speeds up, prompting me to ask something like, "What's going on? You don't need to tell me the content if you don't want to. I just need to know what you need, and if you want to continue the lesson." If the person is feeling unsafe, I do what I can to renew safety in the room; often, simply asking them to look around to see where they are is enough. Beyond that, all of the skills I have are primed to respond to the AT Progression—with the simple key of omniserving the head–spine relationship as the student responds to ideas.

In a group class, the group may play an active role. For instance, they might be the ones who, by their presence, help create safety or may have similar experiences they can relate. The group may also need reassurance from you, the teacher, that all is well, that what is happening is normal. If it seems appropriate, finding a way to lighten the moment is helpful. In a group, you need to find a way to acknowledge what has happened during a turn like this, celebrate it, and move forward. Ideally, the lesson closes with a sustainable plan that reframes the past history constructively and supplies any revealed needs. Not all deeply resonant lessons require this kind of attention—sometimes, they are quite joyous and simple while similarly resonant!

Biopsychosocial wholeness is implicit in every lesson, every turn—and every page of this book.

Part Three

INTEGRATIVE
TEACHING PRACTICE

Chapter 16

DEEP PLAY FACILITATION

In the midst of a workshop, a European training school director suddenly turned around and mildly exclaimed, "No one ever told you the Alexander Technique was hard, did they?" With this question, he illuminated a key value in how I learned and teach the Alexander Technique. While it had never occurred to me to consider this before, my answer to his question was, as you might imagine, "No." A quick glance at any of the videos of Marj's workshops reveals her constant playful perspective. Her living room was an oasis of nonjudgmental, generally joyous exploration. One of her maxims, spoken and lived, was "Learn to laugh at yourself. You always move better with a smile" (Barstow and Brenner 1987, p.37). Even on the occasions when I got frustrated with my progress, my overarching constant was the joy of having this simple, elegant tool in my life.

I borrow the term *deep play* from Diane Ackerman. "Deep play variations" is an apt description of my intended learning environments. From Ackerman: "Above all, play requires freedom. One chooses to play. Play's rules may be enforced, but play is not like life's other dramas. It happens outside ordinary life, and it requires freedom" (Ackerman 1999, p.7). Ackerman, in turn, quotes Dutch historian Johan Huizinga (1872–1945), who was interested in the play element in culture, saying play:

> is an activity which proceeds within certain limits of time and space, in a visible order, according to rules freely accepted, and outside the sphere of necessity or material utility. The play mood is one of rapture and enthusiasm, and is sacred or festive in accordance with the occasion. A feeling of exultation and tension accompanies the action. (Ackerman 1999, p.3)

Stuart Brown, the founder/director of the National Association for Play, whose research includes the biology of play, says, "It is about learning to harness a force that has been built into us through millions of years of evolution, a force that allows us to both discover our most essential selves and enlarge our world" (2009, p.13).

Rather than peripheral to the learning process, play is integral, central. Play has been essential in education throughout human history—from teaching children life skills to developing complicated social structures:

> Play is an activity enjoyed for its own sake. It is our brain's favorite way of learning and maneuvering. Because we think of play as the opposite of seriousness, we don't notice that it governs most of society—political games, in-law games, money games, love games, advertising games, to list only a few spheres where gamesmanship is rampant. (Ackerman 1999, p.11)

Including play in the teaching and learning process cooperates with how humans prefer to learn. Moreover, consciously selected play invites deeper, transformational learning in a nonintrusive way. Play both deepens and lightens learning.

Huizinga's description of play parallels the Alexander Technique's learning environments:

- Classes, workshops, and lessons occur in a chosen environment with a predetermined time limit.

- While the visible order varies from teacher to teacher or circumstance to circumstance, all learning events have a beginning, middle, and end. The teacher and student mutually establish the structure based on the needs of the current moment.

- Teachers and students play by the rules they associate with learning the Alexander Technique. (See following discussion of the rules I believe we use.)

- Alexander Technique learning—as helpful as it might be, and as much as it serves quality, efficiency, and effectiveness, is not necessary or of direct material utility to our survival.

- The mood of lessons varies according to the teachers, students, and circumstances.

- The process of change contains the tension of the choice between an old habitual pattern and a journey to the unknown, and joy is a frequent response to the discovery of new choices. Such joy may appear immediately or over time as the learning process deepens.

Huizinga's definition confirms that every Alexander Technique encounter is play. Experiencing the Alexander Technique as play freed me from concerns about right and wrong, good and bad. I understood that experiments—whatever might happen—were necessary in the journey, to be valued rather than something to be embarrassed about or avoided. Play gave me the courage and willingness to explore, precisely because there were no real-world consequences. The playfulness with which I was taught enabled me to rigorously explore my choices with confidence while receiving constructive, challenging feedback. It is the spirit in which I want to teach.

During one of my sessions about deep play at an international congress, someone said, "Yes, but why *deep play* rather than *play?*" My experience, supported by Ackerman's discussion of deep play versus everyday play, is that deep play occurs when the experience of learning transforms belief, enabling new choices in behavior. Transformation from one whole-self behavior to another chosen, constructive whole-self behavior is the goal of every Alexander Technique encounter. In this sense, every Alexander Technique lesson could be described as "deep," though we all recognize that some discoveries are particularly potent or illuminating. All we can do—for ourselves or for our students—is offer an open invitation to any kind of play, including deep play.

I begin the invitation to play/deep play as I introduce the Alexander Technique, inviting transformation on whatever level is appropriate for that student. My words might be:

We'll be talking today about how your head–spine relationship supports or perhaps gets in the way of what you want to do, as well as how you can learn to choose the quality of that relationship. As we start on this road, I want to offer you some words attributed to A.R. Alexander, the brother of the man who developed this work: "The hallmarks of the Alexander Technique are creativity, spontaneity, and adaptability to change." As we start talking a bit about the head–spine relationship in our coordination, just know that it has implications in all aspects of our lives.

From the first moment of learning, I open the door to deep play, knowing that it may happen that day or in the future.

For the student to play, the teacher must be deep playing. This is something I first learned through the actor–audience relationship in theatre. In the theatre world, if the actor is immersed in specific circumstances and actions while inviting the audience into the story, then the audience's ability to participate and transform is enhanced. If the actor is general in approach, the audience is more likely to watch the performance rather than participate in it. As discussed earlier, we, Alexander Technique teachers, are transforming ourselves as we teach by using the same process while we teach it. Parker Palmer, in considering the vocation of teaching, notes, "We are here not only to transform the world but also to be transformed" (Palmer 2000, p.97). Students are more likely to accept the offer of deep play if they sense and trust that the teacher is already traveling the same pathway.

The students' needs, coordination, and learning processes, as well as the conditions of the day, time, and place—all play roles in how the invitation to learn through play is received. Sometimes, deep play is immediate; sometimes, it occurs over the course of time rather than in a single session. Teachers don't always know when deep play is occurring. Students may reveal what goes on within them during the learning process or keep it private. In my own education, I was often working on issues I didn't reveal to Marj. Since I sometimes ask students to keep journals during their first weeks of study, they may reveal deep play experiences I would otherwise have been oblivious to. One young woman, for instance, often braided her hair in Alexander Technique class. I noted that each lesson, she improved the quality of her coordination. Only after I read her journal did I find out that braiding her hair was a way she devised to heal some deep issues in her relationship with a family member.

Play has structure and rules. The AT Progression provides our structure, our rules. In a space and time designated for teaching/learning Alexander's discoveries, we follow the sequence he offered:

Wanting

Recognizing

Deciding

Gathering Information

Creating a Plan

Asking

Acting/Experimenting (doing the plan)

All of which takes place within the context of freedom of choice.

Structure is a key component in creating the depth of an Alexander Technique play experience, as well as a vital element of creating a safe learning environment. This is "another, very positive feature of play: it creates order, *is* order... Play demands order absolute and supreme. The least deviation from it 'spoils the game'" (Huizinga 1949, p.10; original emphasis). If I stray from this structure when I am teaching, I ask for the group's assent. If, as an example, a performer asks me a question best answered "with my performance coach hat on," then I often literally—and playfully—make the gesture of replacing one invisible hat with another. This signifies that I am now leading from this other role. Maintaining the agreed-upon structure by clearly signaling any deviations from it supports a learning environment that is both challenging and safe. Challenge propels play to deep play. Huizinga supplies that "it is this element of tension and solution that governs all solitary games of skill" (Huizinga 1949, p.11). His definition of tension is uncertainty, movement into the unknown without a guarantee of success—while seeking a solution. The next chapter's discussion of the Alexander Technique in relationship to Ericsson's deliberate practice research investigates the challenge element of play in more depth.

Play researcher Brown says:

> Making all life an act of play occurs when we recognize and accept that there may be some discomfort in play, and that every experience has both pleasure and pain. That is not to say that bliss is suffering. My take is that following your bliss may be difficult, demanding, uncomfortable, tedious at times, but not really suffering... Advanced play, the black belt of play, comes when we realize this and act on it. As long as we are acting in accordance with our central truth, then the outcome will be positive. (Brown 2009, p.205)

As we move forward in our discussion of teaching, we weave the skill threads together toward an integrative practice that plays intelligently with how humans learn best.

Chapter 17

THE RIGOR OF PLAY AND PRACTICE

Play is a rigorous pursuit. Various forms of play have been used to build skills of all kinds, strengths of all kinds, resilience, courage, and willpower in the face of adversity.

In an undergraduate acting class at Penn State, one of my professors—in the midst of a Greek scene study—took us behind the theater building to a small wooded area. He asked us to play tag—with a twist. The person who is "it" closes their eyes and counts to 20 as everyone else hides, then searches for those hiding. When "it" spies someone, they call out that person's name and run to the base; the person who is named also runs to the base, trying to beat "it." If the person gets to base first, they are free; if "it" gets to the base first, the person is caught. Furthermore, if the person beats "it" to the base and people who are already caught are at the base, those people are freed, too. Quite a complicated game. We played for the whole class period, inventing many strategies. We had fun and were deeply invested in each thing we were doing, as well as a wee bit puzzled about how this was acting class. As we gathered at the end of class, our professor said, "If you put half of that commitment into your acting scenes, they would be amazing." Aha! He was giving us clear feedback—and a challenge.

Deep Play as Deliberate Practice

Deep play in the learning environment involves offering challenges and providing skillful feedback. Earlier, I mentioned Anders Ericsson's research on expertise, and the term he coined: *deliberate practice.*

Ericsson's findings shine a light on Alexander Technique teaching practices, particularly related to the role of feedback. Following are the characteristics he identifies as necessary components of deliberate practice, that is, "purposeful practice that knows where it is going and how to get there" (Ericsson and Pool 2016, p.98):

- "Develops skills that other people have already figured out how to do" as well as how to train people to do, guided by a teacher/coach who has experience.

- "Takes place outside one's comfort zone and requires a student to constantly try things that are just beyond his or her current abilities."

- Involves "well-defined, specific goals."

- Requires conscious participation by the student.

- "Involves feedback and modification of efforts in response to feedback."

- "Produces and depends on effective mental representations."

- "Nearly always involves building or modifying previously acquired skills by focusing on particular aspects of those skills and working to improve them specifically; over time this step-by-step improvement will eventually lead to expert performance."

(Ericsson and Pool 2016, pp.99–100)

Following, I discuss Alexander Technique teaching in relationship to each of these principles. This detailed comparison of deliberate practice and the Alexander Technique is intended to reinforce the teaching practices associated with Alexander Technique teaching and learning.

Develops Skills for an Already-"Figured-Out" Process Guided by an Expert

For most of us, our "figured-out" process begins with the teacher we first studied with. In my case, my first Alexander Technique lessons were with Marj. All of our first teachers studied with someone who learned from an expert who spent many hours in practice. Marj was a dancer who went to England to study with F.M. Alexander for a time, then returned to Nebraska. Subsequently, she was in his first training course, then assisted F.M. and A.R. Alexander in Boston from 1934 to 1942. By the time I started studying with her, she had been actively using and teaching the Alexander Technique for many years. She was an expert with a practiced process.

Everyone who teaches this work has such a story because learning to be an Alexander Technique teacher requires committed practice, something akin to my Living Room Étude. The training typically includes not only investigation of your self, but also omniservation of others and teaching of others. We have F.M. Alexander's writings, particularly that first chapter of *The Use of the Self*, as a guide. In addition, we have the writings of many Alexander Technique teachers as well as experts from complementary fields.

While I hold that it must be possible for people to teach themselves the Alexander Technique, and have had the luck of teaching a few people who grasped the work rapidly, we all know that having a teacher guiding us through the process expedites success. Because we learn through our current level of coordination, the way we interpret new information may be skewed by a mistaken belief. In a recent class, even something as simple as a mistaken idea about how the knee moves was preventing someone from walking in the way she wanted to. While the student may have figured this out for herself eventually, my ability as the teacher to question her idea of how knees move enabled her to rapidly alter her walk.

Stretches the Student's Comfort Zone and Requires Resilient Experimentation

At the University of Washington, I teach for the Professional Actor Training Program. It is my one teaching situation in which the students do not directly elect to learn the Alexander Technique. When they join the program, they know Alexander Technique is included, but they don't have a choice if they take the class—it is required. It is also the only situation in which I teach that demands specific progress in a fixed period of time.

In our first class meeting, I acknowledge the incongruity of teaching a class based on freedom of choice while the class is also required.

I give them context for why it is included in their curriculum, and I invite their participation. In the first round of practical experiments, I wait for their "yes." I acknowledge that while they are required to come to class, they do have choice within the class. (Also noting that they actually have choice about whether they come to class, as long as they realize I am required to report their absence, which has consequences.)

All this care in inviting their "yes" is vital because the Alexander Technique asks them to go beyond their comfort zone. In every class. In every exploration. I set up a learning environment that is safe, rich in resources, and full of choice—all in the service of challenging their current conception of themselves and/or their skills. I give them constant, consistent feedback on what they are doing and what might be possible.

Their resilience in experimentation is fueled by my insistence that their own desire leads the lesson—they are willing to explore because they want something. The play-framing of the teaching enhances the pioneering spirit—you can try it out in class before committing to it outside the learning space. While the circumstances of teaching in a required class at a university especially compel care around the "yes," the first request for rigor is to ask these new Alexander Technique students to embrace freedom within a required class.

The Alexander Technique Helps Identify the Learning Edge

The omniservation skills of the Alexander Technique are a tremendous aid in the ability to ascertain where each student's learning edge lives. When I offer an idea, I am endeavoring for what University of California, Los Angeles (UCLA) Psychology Professor Bjorn Bork describes as "finding the sweet spot. There's an optimal gap between what you know and what you're trying to do. When you find that sweet spot, learning takes off" (Coyle 2009, p.19). How a student coordinates to an idea I am offering—specifically, what happens between their head and spine as I offer an idea—gives me a great deal of information as to whether an idea is useful, doable, or sustainable.

One of the reasons I prefer to use my hands to follow my student's return to coordination as a "yes" to the new idea is to watch and listen to them specifically as they enter this "sweet spot." If I am following them when the new idea becomes challenging, then they have more context for saying "yes"—the teacher is signaling that all is well. If we go too far beyond the "sweet spot," then they will stiffen.

When dancers started to tighten between head and spine as they stretched, to challenge the "sweet spot" of their stretch, Marj would invite them to back off a little, then ask themselves to COORDINATE so their heads could move so that all of them could follow so that they could go into the stretch again. If they were unable to sustain their coordination beyond a certain point in the stretch, she'd say something like, "That's enough, you are overstretching." That is, they were trying to go farther than their system could sustain. As soon as they did, they tightened between head and spine and, because the tightening affected the geometry of their whole system, they were no longer stretching the intended muscles, anyway.

Similarly, if a student is working the edges of their "sweet spot," however that manifests in their biopsychosocial self, I offer something similar. If they start to tighten head and spine in the midst of trying out a new idea, we back off, renew the request to coordinate, and try the new idea again. If interference again ensues, we know we have more sleuthing to do, seeking how to refine the message into something doable and ultimately sustainable.

Daniel Coyle's report of his research into talent hotbeds—places where, seemingly inexplicably, many people seemed expert in a particular skill—revealed (similar to Ericsson) a process guided by a gifted teacher. He calls the process "deep practice," which he considers essentially equivalent to Ericsson's deliberate practice (Coyle 2009, p.51) "Deep practice...involves a cycle of distinct actions. 1. Pick a target. 2. Reach for it. 3. Evaluate the gap between the target and the reach. 4. Return to step one" (Coyle 2009, p.92). What the Alexander Technique offers is a crucial tool in step three so that the return to the first step—the stretch into the skill level just beyond comfort—is informed by how each person's coordination is responding to the ideas.

Coyle's steps in deep practice mirror the AT Progression. To pick a target (step one) requires a desire for a target, one that you recognize you aren't reaching, and a decision to go for it. Reaching for it the first time (step two) gathers information. From this information, the evaluation results in the creation of a new plan (step three). The new plan is used to reach again (step four).

The Alexander Technique teacher's ability to omniserve the subtlety of how the head–spine relationship responds to nuanced new ideas is a valuable aid in becoming what Coyle calls a "talent whisperer." Another virtue of such a teacher is perceptiveness: "on the macro level, the coaches I met approached new students with the curiosity of an investigative reporter... And on the microlevel, they constantly monitored the student's reaction to their coaching, checking whether their message was being absorbed" (Coyle 2009, p.185).

What he calls perceptiveness, I would categorize as an omnis-ervation skill, the same one I learned in Marj's living room, an essential skill in guiding students to that area just outside their comfort zone, where learning flourishes.

Specific Goals

Receiving information about the students' desires is particularly important because they usually have specific goals. Lessons ideally center around student goals. As a teacher, I may need to negotiate some intermediate and specific steps on the way to the larger goal (in Alexander Technique language, the "means-whereby"). Generally, the goal can be stated as the ability to sustain a dynamic, coordinated head–spine relationship in order to do the task. "Once an overall goal has been set, a teacher or coach will develop a plan for making a series of small changes that will add up to the desired larger change" (Ericssson and Pool 2016, p.99). This aspect of deliberate practice is particularly key, for success in the intermediate steps rewards the excursion outside the comfort zone and fuels continued deep and deliberate practice.

The Student Consciously Participates

Virtually every page of this book emphasizes this point: using the Alexander Technique requires conscious volition from the student.

The Teacher-Student Conversation– Feedback and Response

Again, the elements for working in the "sweet spot" just beyond the comfort zone: the teacher uses omniservation skills to guide students in the direction of their desire, offering ideas, followed by experimentation, followed by feedback leading to new experiments; these iterations continue. As noted, the Living Room Étude taught me many of the skills I needed for this. Another occasional practice in Marj's workshops also helped develop these skills.

Marj would invite the group to divide into smaller groups, then begin a conversation. Innocently, we started talking to each other, wondering what she was planning. She would ask us to pause, then say, "Now, talk to each other about what you noticed about yourself while you were talking." We shared with each other either what we noticed or the fact that we hadn't been paying attention to ourselves. She asked us to pause again. "Now, talk to each other about what you noticed about each other while you were talking." At first, this seemed an impossible task—how could I use the Alexander Technique to talk and be able to report what I was doing while also being able to report what my student was doing? At some point, I realized that what I thought of as an impossible task was exactly the skill I needed for teaching.

This beautiful practice—I would call it an Alexander Technique game—was significant in that it also taught me to be the "hawk eye" Coyle talks about without causing undue tightening in my student. I learned how to describe what I was seeing in my fellow conversationalists in a way that didn't elicit a tightening response from them. And, if I did see head–spine interference as I said something, I had the opportunity to rephrase what I was saying.

Through this game as well as other experiences, I learned to be rigorous and challenging in my feedback in a way that elicited interest, curiosity, and excitement in my students. The variations of these teaching conversations are endless. At the point of writing this chapter, I paid attention to all the ways I was offering feedback and responding to see what I could generalize. Beyond the skills we explored in Part Two of this book, all I came up with was whole-self listening and whole-self responding. The range of what I was drawing on (we'll talk about this in Chapter 18) was large; each person is unique.

Effective Mental Representations

What Ericsson calls "effective mental representations" parallels F.M. Alexander's conceptions of belief and psychophysical history.

What the feedback loop often reveals is the need for an update in these representations. A simple example of this is: if your students believe that the head–spine relationship is in a different place than it actually is, their self-representation affects their ability to use F.M. Alexander's discovery. When their image of themselves becomes more accurate, their ability to use Alexander Technique grows. It is surprising how often an anatomical misconception is significant in a lesson. Studying our human design so that you have the knowledge to address these misconceptions is beneficial. In addition, the more you know, the more you are able to omniserve and analyze.

These conceptions can include all aspects of who we are and the world we have grown up in. I have had students who realized that their tightening was a result of attempting literally to become invisible. And I'll never forget someone who was breathing like their favorite childhood cartoon character—who had a rather peculiar breathing pattern!

At the moment of head–spine tightening as someone says something, a skillful question might reveal the whole-self representation that needs an update:

> over time this step-by-step improvement will eventually lead to expert performance. (Ericsson and Pool 2016, p.100)

This sounds like every Alexander Technique encounter, whether with myself, a student, or many students.

Chapter 18

THE INTEGRATED SELF IS CREATIVE

Some years ago, when a friend asked me to sit on a panel about creativity, my first task was to answer the question, "How do I define creativity?" What emerged was a metaphor that has stuck with me—creativity is an open-doorways dance with all of me talking to all of me in response to a need or desire. Any and all bits of my knowledge and experience are welcome to dance in any combination with any of my other knowledge/ experience bits. Learning the Alexander Technique exponentially enhanced my integrative process and, therefore, my creativity.

My identification of myself as creative began long before my Alexander Technique training. My father called me Sarah sometimes as a baby because apparently my behavior reminded him of Sarah Bernhardt. An early creative memory comes from middle school. The assignment was to draw a picture about Christmas. Art was not my best subject in school. (And, yes, I have used Alexander Technique to change my relationship to drawing.) I ruminated on this assignment— and vividly remember the moment I thought, "Three kings, triangles have three sides—I could create a whole picture of triangles." Using color was something I did okay, but I just couldn't get the shapes the way I wanted them; luckily, a ruler solved my problem. I am reliving my excitement even as I write this; and the art teacher was properly encouraging!

I believe that creativity is our birthright. If we didn't learn to divide ourselves into separate segments, then creativity would flow automatically. I hear a lot of folks who don't identify as creative. Perhaps this is because their definition of *creativity* is narrow; perhaps it is because their coordination closes doorways between different aspects of their experience/knowledge so the dance that creates new ideas is less active. Countless times I have seen creativity emerge as coordination improves.

Teaching the Alexander Technique is a tool to opening those doorways to all aspects of our biopsychosocial selves. In my first book for performers, I proffered a variety of ways in which the Alexander Technique facilitates creativity:

- When our instrument functions optimally, our ability to imagine alternate possibilities "suddenly" reappears. In many lessons I have taught, the solution to a problem emerges at the same time as the student's coordination improves.

- Constructive thinking is by its nature creative, constructing/building a new concept, theory, idea.

- Learning the Alexander Technique cultivates curiosity.

- "So that" as the linking clause in the representation of the AT Progression opens doors in a continuum. (Rather than "and" which would separate the rooms.)

(Madden 2014, pp.279–287)

In considering creativity in the teaching process, I offer in Table 18.1 a side-by-side comparison of the characteristics Mihaly Csikszentmihalyi reports as constants in an enjoyable flow experience, the Alexander Technique, and Ericsson's deliberate practice traits.

Table 18.1 Comparing Creativity, the Alexander Technique, and Deliberate Practice

Creativity (Csikszentmihalyi 1996, pp.110–113)	Alexander Technique	Deliberate Practice (Ericsson and Pool 2016, pp.99–100)
Clear goals every step of the way.	Wanting.	Has well-defined goals.
Immediate feedback to one's actions.	Feedback from the teacher, or from the activity the Alexander Technique is being used to do.	Has feedback and response to feedback.
A balance between challenge and skills.	The teacher and student work together to build skills incrementally.	The task is just outside the skill level, or "comfort zone."

Creativity (Csikszentmihalyi 1996, pp.110–113)	Alexander Technique	Deliberate Practice (Ericsson and Pool 2016, pp.99–100)
Action and awareness are merged.	Using the researched and selected plan to do the chosen activity. (Gathering information, creating a plan, asking yourself to carry out the plan.)	Requires full attention and conscious choice.
Distractions are excluded from consciousness.	I would reframe this: Focus is chosen, rather than distractions excluded.	Not mentioned.
No worry about failure.	The play atmosphere of the learning environment supports a "failure is part of the learning" perspective.	Making mistakes and responding to them is the expectation, so the learning "game" is about development rather than right and wrong.
Self-consciousness disappears.	The play atmosphere of the learning environment encourages focus on process.	Requires focus, which eliminates self-consciousness.
The sense of time becomes distorted.	This may occur, but is not necessarily part of the process. Certainly, Alexander Technique students and teachers are frequently surprised that the time has gone by so quickly.	Not mentioned.
The activity becomes autotelic (he describes this as "enjoying it for its own sake").	The play atmosphere of the learning environment, along with the increasing skill of the student, tend to create this sort of enjoyment.	Learning tasks are selected so that incremental improvement can be appreciated. While Ericsson notes that some aspects of deliberate practice are not "enjoyable," my experience is that when the lesson is framed by the student's desire, the effort towards it is enjoyable. Brown's assessment, cited in Chapter 16, that play has significant challenge, but is ultimately pleasurable, matches my experience.

The Alexander Technique could be described as a creative process, learned through deliberate practice. As teachers, we both enable creativity and engage in a creative process. When we are teaching, if we are embracing the open doorways of creativity, omniservational information from and about our students, along with all of our learning and experience, are dancing with each other, forming and reforming ideas in service of the learning need. A template for that process could be:

> I use the Alexander Technique
> So that I can omniserve my students
> As I invite them to be with me while I am with them
> So that I can gather information from many sources
> (*including the Alexander Technique, what I know about anatomy, what activity they are doing, the environment we are in, and so forth*)
> So that I can create a plan
> (*taking information from multiple sources, and through the lens of the Alexander Technique, creating a plan, linking images / ideas to respond to the student's needs, wants, desires*)
> So that I can invite the student to explore using the plan
> (*using the Alexander Technique for any of the many ways I might teach*)

Teaching requires the ability to link images in new ways. As with all skills, this takes practice.

At the University of Washington, I began using the Alexander Technique in relationship to creativity skills when I saw some actors consistently diminishing their coordination when asked to play in imaginary circumstances. The story of my original observations and subsequent hypothesis is covered in more detail in my article, "Refurbishing images in actors and others" in *Direction* (Madden 2005, pp.9–12). What developed from my omniservations were whole-self-pathways-to-imagination exercises—creativity-specific practices. The exercises rely on the Alexander Technique's ability to coordinate the whole individual; they also draw from actor training exercises, studies in neuroscience, and nature.

When I presented a workshop on creativity at the International Congress of Alexander Technique Teachers in Limerick in 2015, the group had an epiphany as they discovered one of these exercises developed for actors was an essential skill for teaching:

Use the Alexander Technique to link three images–sustaining your coordination in a metaphorical thinking process.

In this practice, we combine three different concrete stimuli in a one-sentence story (ideally, without *and*, *or*, or other connectives). An example of three images might be book, rose, and maple leaf. A one-sentence "story" might go "We found a rose when we opened the book to press the maple leaf." (An example of a nonlinked sentence would be "I was carrying a book and saw a rose and picked up a maple leaf.")

Every option that appears as you play with these three images is fine—it isn't about the success of combining, but about the effort towards it. For acting and teaching purposes, it is ideal to use the Alexander Technique to think of the sentence while inviting people to be with you while you are with them as you wonder how to bring the images together. This is a game I teach to classes when the exploration centers on the thinking and/or imagination process.

Sustaining coordination as we link images is exactly what we need for teaching: bringing together students' wants and ideas with our own information. Playing the "link three images" game is something you can practice anytime, anywhere—waiting in lines, walking down the street, and so on, and so forth.

Chapter 19

PREPARING FOR TEACHING

Teaching Readiness

The questions I use to analyze the circumstances of a lesson also guide my preparation for teaching. Sometimes my self-research is relatively informal. I might, for instance, review my circumstances while walking from my car to the classroom. For new teaching circumstances, or specialized ones, I may prepare for weeks, perhaps even months. (When I was a topic keynote speaker for the Freiburg International Congress, for instance, I readied myself for the task for almost a year.) Reviewing my answers to the following questions periodically keeps me up to date with myself, my new knowledge, and my changing perspectives.

Aspects of this analysis are key to creating the different types of class structures detailed in the ensuing chapters. The questions, framed specifically for teaching readiness, are as follows.

People Questions

Who am I?

Who am I with?

If it is a group, what do I know about the group?

What is significant about my relationships with the group?

Learning Environment Questions

Where am I teaching?

What time of day am I teaching?

What resources are available to me?

Which other people or objects might be around?

What is significant to me about the learning environment?

Desire Questions

What do I want? Personally? Professionally?

It is useful to examine what you want in increments beginning with "What do I want right now?" and progressing to "What do I want for my life?"

Is anything in my way?

Action Question

What am I doing or planning to do to get what I want?

How the Questions Empower You
People Questions

Opening the doorways of resources, confidence, honesty, knowledge, and creativity begins as I answer the questions about myself. I am constantly surprised by how often some seemingly auxiliary piece of information from a seemingly unrelated aspect of my life helps me unlock a moment in a lesson. Once, as I looked at how an actor was holding a script:

Me: Do you ride horses?

Actor: (*surprised*) Yes.

Me: You are holding that script like you are holding the reins on your horse and trying to prevent the horse from pulling the reins through your fingers. I don't think the script is going to pull on you.

Actor: (*still surprised, while releasing the grip on the script*) How did you know?

Me: I have taught the Alexander Technique to dressage riders and recognized the way you had your hand organized.

When thoroughly answering the question "Who am I?" you fill many pages, and it is worth doing such an extensive listing every so often. My list might include (in no particular order): Alexander Technique teacher, acting teacher, director, mother, daughter, cat owner, jazz dance-skilled, university lecturer, ice-skating devotee, crocheter, speaker of some French/German/Swiss German and a little Japanese, author, childbirth educator...

Your students have similar lists. While you will never know their comprehensive list, considering what you do know is useful preparation. A student's knowledge in one field may contribute to constructive planning for a seemingly unrelated activity. One performer, for instance, asked to bring his golf clubs to class. I was stunned because, when he held a golf club, his coordination was amazing. Calling on his golfing coordination helped him in all of his activities. Conversely, one surgeon thought her arms were hurting from computer work, but discovered what was actually in her way was that she always held her arms as she needed to in a sterile field getting ready to operate. If I hadn't known she was a surgeon, I might not have recognized the pattern I was seeing.

When teaching groups, your resource list is enriched by the knowledge and experience of everyone in the room. You want to set things up so that each individual feels welcome to contribute.

The "What is significant..." question acknowledges any relationships that are part of the biopsychosocial event of the class. From people taking a friend along with them for a first lesson to someone considering adding Alexander Technique to a company's training program, acknowledging the significance of their relationship to you is a key step in optimally preparing yourself. If you know that someone has a medical background, you might choose to use more technical vocabulary; if you know someone is new, you might be attentive to explaining shorthand; if you know someone is an expert in a field and a question comes up about that field, you might solicit ideas from them.

Learning Environment Questions

Beyond the details mentioned in Chapter 4, is this space significant to you in any way? Every room I teach in at Hutchinson Hall at the University of Washington is rich with stories and significance both for me and for the students in the room. Nearly every spot contains a teaching story. When I did a workshop for the university where I was first introduced to the Alexander Technique, my relationship to the students was enriched: I realized, "One of them could be me." When I prepared to teach at the Carrington Hotel in Katoomba, Australia, and realized it was possible that F.M. Alexander might once have been there, I felt a sense of gratitude. If you are visiting a new school or one that has just moved, that first time there is special, and celebrating the new place might be part of the workshop. It works the other way around, too: a particular room where I teach regularly is not one I would choose as a teaching space; preparing to teach there requires me to consciously renew my desire to teach, particularly noting that the desire to teach is stronger than my dislike of the room. Once I have prepared, the room is no longer an obstacle.

Desire Questions

Just as our students' learning experience begins with desire, our desire leads our steps into the teaching room. As with the question "Who am I?" this question ("What do I want?") is worth doing in depth periodically, and, again, it is one I do both informally as I walk to class, and formally when the occasion calls for it.

When considering the formal answer, begin with what you want right at the moment you ask the question. Continue incrementally through what you want for the next ten minutes, the next hour, the length of the class, the day, the week, the month, the season, and so on, until you arrive at "What do you want for your life?"

People sometimes ask why the question "Is anything in your way?" is on the list. Their concern is that bringing this up is somehow nonconstructive, rather preferring to ignore it. Unfortunately, like not scratching an itch, ignoring obstacles tends to make them bigger obstacles. The teaching room I just mentioned is an example. Being honest about your obstacles gives you the opportunity to take care of them through a constructive plan. Note that obstacles are not always "heavy" issues—sometimes, the obstacle is simply that you are tired.

Action Question

Synthesizing the answers to your preparatory questions augments your action plan for teaching, assisting you in considering which of the many ways you might teach are applicable to your current situation. The remainder of Part Three is dedicated to explicating many Alexander Technique teaching variations.

Why It Matters

The Alexander Technique facilitates coordination in whatever you are doing; it doesn't discriminate between plans that are constructive and efficient and those that are less optimal. It helps us do either one better. We still tighten on those less optimal plans, but we'll tighten better.

Some Examples of How Preparation Has Helped Me

One teaching day got extra full: I started around 8 a.m., and my last class finished at 9 p.m. A long-time student had some friends in town for the day and had asked me to teach them. I had agreed, so they were going to arrive soon for a 9:15 lesson. I was exhausted and feeling reluctant, and yet I knew I needed to find freedom to choose. "Who am I?" revealed a teacher who wanted to keep her word. "Who am I teaching?" revealed a relationship to my current student as well as respect for the people who wanted the lesson. "What time is it?" reminded me that it was a limited time commitment. "Are there any obstacles?" elicited a promise to myself that, in the future, I would schedule lessons before 9 p.m. I went on to enjoy teaching the lessons that night.

I was teaching a breakout group in a larger workshop. As the organizer was assigning groups, he said, "I'm putting Cathy in that group because she is good at handling anger." I had already done my prep; suddenly, I had a new obstacle to deal with—it hadn't occurred to me to expect anger. I reviewed my "Who am I?" which now included his assessment of my skills. I renewed my desire to teach and called upon my back-pocket plan for responding to the unexpected, particularly anger: I use the Alexander Technique to invite people to be with me while I am with them as I gather the information I need to respond to the needs of the student and the group. I also redid the three-step prep that I will discuss later. I was glad I had renewed all of my prep; I needed it, as someone in my group did get very angry (all worked out well).

When I was invited to do a talk for the managers of a large corporation, I had been answering these questions over several weeks while preparing the workshop content. As I walked from the parking lot to the building, I reviewed my answers because I felt I needed one more piece of information. When I asked myself, "Who am I teaching?" I found what I needed: these managers would have a lot of similarity to my father. Having this bit of information helped me to establish rapport as I began the session.

Preparing for big events sometimes takes months. As a Congress Teacher for the International Congress in Sydney, knowing I was representing Marj and her work, it took me a long while to deeply explore my "Who am I?" so I could teach clearly as myself. The exploration led me to realize that what would take care of my obstacle was to plan clearly what I wanted to teach. Because I prefer to teach based on student desire, yet I wouldn't know who my students were until they walked into the room, I was puzzled about how to plan. I decided to prepare for as many kinds of classes and topics as I could. I created a notebook full of class plans and resources, inventing ways to offer choices to the groups as I began each session. Some of the topics included: Beginner's Mind, The Power of "I Don't Know," Groups, Andragogy, How Do You Teach Without Making Someone Wrong? Games as a Teaching Tool, Creating a Learning Series with Games, and Simplicity. My notebook included quotes from F.M. Alexander and other experts. Once I had assembled my personal teaching resource, I no longer felt hampered by concerns of unworthiness to represent Marj. I was ready to represent myself, the teacher I had become through my study with Marj.

Right Before

Csikszentmihalyi notes that most creative individuals have determined a set of patterned activities that prepare them most effectively for their work: "what matters most is that we shape the immediate surroundings, activities, and schedules so as to feel in harmony with the small segment of the universe where we happen to be located" (1996, p.146).

The teaching playground is a sacred place. I want to prepare in such a way that I bring all of my resources to bear while also identifying what is personal. Consequently, I do have a patterned practice before entering that playground: using the Alexander Technique to do a three-step sequence that includes a personal inventory, a sensory exploration, and an active gratitude exploration (Madden 2014, pp.239–240). This practice acknowledges what is happening with me in the moment so I can leave outside the teaching space anything I need to leave. It wakes up my senses for omniservation. It actively invites a constructive frame of mind. Because I practice this sequence regularly, in addition to preparing me for teaching, it signals me that I am about to engage in a specialized, sacred task.

Chapter 20

PLANNING FOR TEACHING

When someone first asked me how I plan a workshop or a class, I had to research my process and analyze it. Both surprisingly and not surprisingly, I discovered I was using the AT Progression in a slightly different variation:

Wanting: I gather the wants of the class, as well as my own wants.

Recognizing: I recognize that I want to create an environment where we can address/learn about the wants expressed.

Deciding: I decide to plan.

Gathering Information: The wants are my first piece of information. Other information includes the preparatory questions such as who is coming, where we are, and how much time we have. I also draw upon my knowledge of the Alexander Technique and related fields. Depending on how far in advance I am in planning, this may also be a moment to do some research.

Creating a Plan: I design a beginning, middle, and end, knowing I have the freedom to make other choices.

Acting/Experimenting: I teach (*always knowing I have the freedom of choice to teach or not teach*).

Using the same process to design the class that I use to coordinate myself while teaching it to others gives another layer of depth, of resonance, to the process.

How I Use These Steps to Plan
Wanting

Our students arrive with a desire to learn the Alexander Technique for the same reasons research says adults generally come to learn. They experience a need in their life—more skill, more competency, a desire to achieve their full potential in some way. They are in class for themselves (Knowles *et al.* 2005, p.159).

I always assume that if they are in class, then they want to be there. For a course that requires registration, they may have already expressed their wishes. Even if I have already asked them, I talk with them about why they are there as they arrive for class. Their needs may have shifted. This happened just the other day: a new student arrived; I had reviewed her e-mail and planned how I would introduce the Alexander Technique to her. As I said, "You said you wanted to work on walking and..." before I finished my sentence, she interrupted, "I don't know why I wrote that; my neck hurts all the time, that is what I want to work on."

I learned how important it is to reconfirm student desire on the beach in Brittany. My friend and colleague Rosa Luisa Rossi and I had sent out an invitation for an Alexander Technique and Arts workshop. We had carefully prepared a detailed daily schedule, leading to a final performance. As we gathered on the beach the first evening, sitting on large stones and hearing the rolling waves, we invited everyone to say who they were and why they were there. We listened in amazement, and a bit of shock. Not one of the participants was there for the workshop we had advertised. *Not one!* That evening, we redesigned the course.

When I meet a class for the first time, I plan an opening activity to "wake up" their wants. A common choice is the paper art project described in "Games Digest" that becomes their nametag. On the back side of their artwork, I ask them to write why they are there. With this, before I ask them to share their wishes with the group, they will have thought about how to word their request. Particularly in an introductory class, I assure everyone that answers like "My friend told me to come" and "I just want to know what it is" are perfectly fine.

Whether I collect these wants before or as I see the student, I am listening for common threads in the students' requests, to consider if there might be a useful sequencing of the lessons, as I omniserve how they are moving as they say what they want. If I have planned a sequence for the class, I consider how what I planned and am hearing match or don't match. Sometimes, *want* is a loaded word for people because, in their biopsychosocial history, it wasn't okay to want something. In this case, other versions of the question such as "What brought you here today?" or "What is the next step on your journey?" might elicit the information you need in a way that means they can respond.

When the Want Needs to Be Nurtured

Because I teach an undergraduate class at a university during Summer Term, I have occasionally had people come to class simply because it was the right number of credits at the right time of day. One student registered because his name was Alexander. My summer course is a one-week intensive in the evening, so people sometimes sign up for it only because it fits their schedule and fulfills an arts requirement. One year, several business majors registered. They didn't know what they had signed up for. I remember asking one of them while teaching him the first night, "What are you thinking?" He said, quite honestly, "I wonder what I am doing here." Each day, I found ways to elicit desire from him, often by offering choices: "Do you want to review what we did yesterday or would you like to experiment with something else, perhaps reaching for something?" He would pick an activity and hung in with the class and the reading. I knew he had turned a corner when, on the last night, he brought his track shoes and asked for a lesson about running.

The other time I am extra attentive to the want is when someone comes to a lesson because a friend or relative has sent them. Most of the time this works quite easily. Occasionally, they have arrived solely to appease their referrer, rather than because they want to be there. My job then becomes to invite them to the work by providing the information they need to select it for themselves. Again, this generally works well, partially because I acknowledge the circumstance and let them know it's okay with me if they don't like it.

Recognizing and Deciding

My overall arc of recognition begins at the point where I decide to teach the particular lesson, class, workshop, or residential. As I hear what people want, I recognize that I want to create the conditions for each individual to express their desire as the first step in learning what they want to learn. Their recognition is in action from the moment they sign up.

I decide that I am willing to walk with them in their learning journey. This is a step I don't take lightly. Not that it is hard, but rather a key understanding that while I have experienced meeting new Alexander Technique students many times, this is a first moment for them. I respect this moment of choice—the first walk into the teaching studio.

Gathering Information and Creating a Plan

Specific details on these steps are part of the discussion in the ensuing chapters. Some general thoughts follow, noting that some classes involve a more informal planning while others are intricate projects.

A quick example of informal planning: I have a small workshop tomorrow; I know who is coming and generally what their interests are. We have several hours, and I am wondering if I want to bring in something specific or wait for their questions. My primary preparation is to think of them. Everyone coming has studied with me for a while and is in some stage of learning to teach or continuing teacher education. By morning, I expect to have a specific idea "ready" because I have learned that what works for me in planning is to gather all the information, wonder what would be appropriate, and give myself some time for the ideas to percolate. (Consequently, whenever I can, I plan early.) In this case, I specifically set up to create an overnight "percolation." This is also my plan for multiple-day workshops: I gather lots of information, and make the plan when I wake up in the morning. Part of the process is answering the preparatory questions from Chapter 19. (Quick report on the previous example: I had an idea for the class, and never needed it. They arrived and started asking questions immediately.)

Acting/Experimenting

The class, lesson, or workshop is when the planning progression moves into action and experimentation. The next chapter, "The Turn," and ensuing chapters offer a profusion of possibilities for carrying out the teaching plan.

Planning Guidelines

To review, as we head into planning for specific teaching scenarios, here are some general ideas that infuse my process:

- Honesty and kindness.

- The AT Progression chart.

- Is it constructive? Possible? Within my control? Ecological?

- Knowles/Clarke andragogy (adult learning) principles (Knowles *et al.* 2005; Clarke 1998).

- Do I have a variety of ways of presenting the material to appeal to many different learning styles?

- Play. Because F.M. Alexander sometimes called his process "the work," Stuart Brown's words on work and play are apt: "The quality that work and play have in common is creativity. In both we are building our world, creating new relationships, neural connections, objects… Most important, true play that comes from our own inner needs and desires is the only path to finding lasting joy and satisfaction in our work" (Brown 2009, p.127).

When I reviewed Jean Illsley Clarke's Planning Wheel, its similarity to what I have presented—beginning with the preparation for teaching and using the AT Progression to design classes—became apparent. I offer it side by side with the steps we have been discussing because, as andragogic specialists say, alternative ways of viewing an idea aids learning (Table 20.1).

Table 20.1 Clarke Planning Wheel Adapted for the Alexander Technique

Jean Illsley Clarke Planning Wheel, adapted for the Alexander Technique (Clarke 1998, p.104)	Alexander Technique teaching
1. What values guide your teaching of Alexander Technique?	My values arise from my perspective on the Alexander Technique.
2. What do you want as you teach this group? In general?	My perspective on the Alexander Technique and why I teach it, as well as what I want to teach this specific group.

3. What specific goals do you have for this class/workshop/lesson?	My "fancy" description of Alexander Technique answers this question for me: constructive conscious kindness to yourself, cooperating with your design, supporting your desires and dreams. As I consider specific groups and students, particular goals appear.
4. What is your action plan for the class? What resources do you have/need?	From gathering information, I create a plan for action.
5. Teach the class.	Creating the conditions in which students can learn what they want to learn, with my intention to walk with them as they learn.
6. Gather information from how the class went to use for future planning.	Gathering information, always and continually.

Beginning, Middle, and End

As I plan the structure of the class, the framework for the learning playground follows Aristotle's description of story:

> A whole is something that has a beginning, a middle, and an end. A beginning is an item that does not itself follow necessarily upon something else, but which has some second item following necessarily upon it. Conversely, an end is an item that naturally follows, either necessarily or commonly, upon something else, but has nothing following it. A middle is an item that both follows upon a preceding item and has another item following upon itself. (Aristotle 2013, p.26)

Whatever template I may be using to guide my planning—AT Progression, Clarke's process, a deliberate practice model, or something else—everything fits into the container of a beginning, middle, and end. A key element of creating a space for deep play is the cognizance of the time boundary.

In Alexander Technique learning events of whatever kind, the beginning includes the invitation to be part of a learning community characterized by a nonjudgmental, playful atmosphere, and an initial agreement on the content through gathering information about wants, desires, or needs. The middle uses the AT Progression to deliberately develop and practice studied rehearsed plans that respond to the wants/desires/needs expressed. The end empowers the participants to continue deliberate practice in the world. In ensuing chapters focusing on a variety of learning events, beginnings, middles, and ends are the guiding organizational tool.

Chapter 21

THE TURN

Already mentioned frequently, "the turn" could be described as the central unit of any Alexander Technique learning event. It typically refers to the time when an individual and the teacher are working together to answer a specific question or examine a particular activity. It is a discrete unit with an identifiable beginning, middle, and end. While I have emphasized that teaching a turn within a group class is always teaching everyone, the focus is on the individual who asks the question. Calling it a "turn" probably grew out of the game play element of turns taken in sequence.

Actual transcripts of lessons are inappropriate; a lesson is a personal journey. And most lessons include a great deal of shorthand language and nonverbal communication. A turn I taught yesterday had about five minutes of talking, in which neither one of us actually finished our sentence. We'd start to say something, then her coordination changed, leading to a new question—over and over again, faster than we could complete a recognizable sentence. What I offer here instead is a series of fictional turns in which I use complete sentences and describe nonverbal interaction. These are composites of turns I have taught—imaginary, yet based in reality. My intention is to open a window into the moment-to-moment interactions of teaching. These sessions presume a student generally conversant with the AT Progression.

Student One

She attends a weekly class. While she found out about Alexander Technique through the world of theatre because she is an actress, her explorations more often relate to her day job.

Turn One

Teacher: Who has something they'd like to explore?

Student: I've got a question about work. I get such a headache every day.

> *Not surprisingly, as she starts to talk about this, she tightens between head and spine such that her spine is pressed back and her shoulder blades are pulled toward her spine in the back.*

Teacher: That's tough…what is your job? What kinds of things are you doing?

Student: I am the receptionist in a law office. I answer the phone, greet people, and transcribe interviews when I am not busy with those tasks.

> *I note that Student is tightening more as she talks about transcribing interviews, which leads to the next question.*

Teacher: Is there a particular part of the job that you think might be the culprit?

Student: (*pause*) I think it might be the transcription…I just get so nervous when I do it.

> *I note the emotional information. "Nervous" is an ambiguous description. I probably need to ask a question to clarify since there's no way to know exactly what Student means. I'm guessing that it might be about "getting things right" or perhaps speed, but it could be simply that she is tightening while transcribing and the tightening itself is causing the emotional response. My first plan is to "mock up" Student's workplace to get more information.*

Teacher: Let's set up something like your work situation and see what is happening. What do you need?

> *Student describes her workspace and I enlist the help of the rest of the class to set things up; one student offers their laptop, another has ear buds, and a third enjoys a bit of fun decorating the desk so that it looks like a workspace. I offer Alexander Technique quick turns to people as they make up the office. Once the desk is set up, the turn continues.*

Teacher: Okay, decide you are transcribing, and… (*seeing tightening as soon as Student moves her arms*) Let's pause a second and look at that first movement.

Student: Yeah, I tightened as soon as I started to move.

Teacher: What if you ask to COORDINATE so that your head can move so that all of you can follow so that you can look at the computer?

> *As Student asks herself to coordinate, I am using my hands to follow her as she changes as a "yes" to the new idea.*

Teacher: Great, now continue to ask yourself to COORDINATE so that your head can move so that all of you can follow so that you can look at your hands and then move them to the keyboard.

> *As Student continues asking herself, I continue to use my hands to follow as a "yes" to the new idea. When the student's hands are almost to the keyboard, Student tightens again, similar to the tightening she exhibited when she was talking earlier about transcribing. The timing of the tightening seems to correspond with when she would have needed a slight movement at the sternoclavicular joint. At that point, instead of using front muscles to move the arm forward, she collapses her torso toward the back, a version of the slump, and starts to use less appropriate muscles to move the arm.*

Teacher: What did you notice?

> *Visually, I include the whole room in this question, inviting the whole group to consider what they saw.*

Student: As I started to move my arms forward, I suddenly tightened overall.

Teacher: Would everyone please point to the only bone-to-bone joint of the arm to the body?

> *Everyone points, some to the sternoclavicular joint, some to the glenohumeral joint, most to a point between the two. Student is pointing to a point between the two. In pointing out how many different ideas are in the room, I note that this particular arm joint is a surprise to most people, hopefully assuaging any concerns for anyone who pointed to a "wrong" place.*

Teacher: Let's take a look at some anatomy.

I spend some time with the whole group looking at various anatomy books and a skeleton. The group also experiments with different arm movements. Note: I prefer to use medical texts for my anatomy references in class. When I use an Alexander Technique anatomy book, even if the representations are well done, people could get the impression that Alexander anatomy is somehow different from regular anatomy.

(*to Student*) Do you want to see what happens if you use the Alexander Technique to move to the computer with your new arm information?

Student: Sure.

Teacher: Great, and anyone who wants to can experiment along with us—we all spend a good bit of time at computers.
      Ask yourself to COORDINATE so that your head can move so that all of you can follow so that you can look at your hands and then move them to the keyboard.

I am using touch to communicate at the start of the movement, but take my hands away as Student takes over and successfully gets to the keyboard.

Student: That is so different.

Teacher: What flavor of different?

Student: It feels really easy but I totally think I am hunched over and slumpy.

She doesn't look this way; she looks poised for movement, and her arms have a lot less pressure in them.

Teacher: (*to the group*) Does she look slumpy?

The group feedback is important because, from Student's intonation, she cares about whether she is slumpy in relationship to the outside world. The group in the room can reassure her that they would not judge her that way.

Group: "She looks totally upright." "I felt slumpy in my lesson, too—I see what you were explaining to me." "She looks a lot easier." "She looked like she was fighting herself before, now the movement is simpler."

Teacher: I have a suspicion that the way you were moving your arms might be what's causing the headaches. It was causing extra tightening in a region that is a known culprit in use-related headaches. Do you want to try that out this week and see what happens?

I know that the question about nervousness has not been addressed and choose not to bring it back up. The topic has disappeared over the course of the lesson. Student has been smiling, laughing, enjoying the learning.

Student: Yes.

Teacher: What's great is that you have a cue to remind you. When it is time to do the transcription, you can use this process each time. How would you describe what you are doing?

Student: I ask myself to COORDINATE so that my head can move so that all of me can follow…

Student is moving as she speaks while I watch. She stops speaking and I wait for a moment.

Teacher: So that…?

Student looks puzzled.

Teacher: Remember that it needs to be connected to what you are doing.

Student: Oh…right! I ask myself to COORDINATE so that my head can move so that all of me can follow so that I can look at my hands as I move them to the keyboard.

Student makes the action as she speaks and I see that she is carrying through the new idea successfully. Student even notices when she starts to go back to the old plan and, without prompting, returns to the new plan herself. I recognize Student's success and deem it the appropriate moment to bring the lesson to a close. My hope is always to end a turn on a successful sustainable moment of learning.

Teacher: Great, and that was a nice renewal of your plan midway through. You can let us know next week how it went. Does anyone else have any omniservations or questions about this lesson?

Turn Two

It's one week later. During the time right before class, a slightly social time as I offer quick walks to everyone while they arrive, I check in with Student about her headaches. She says she's been experimenting with the transcription and it seemed better, but every time she had to go to work, the headache appeared midmorning. I ask her if she wants to take another turn with her day job as her activity to see if we could get another clue about what was happening. I note Student saying "had to" and wonder if how she is thinking about work is the problem. Later in the class, Student volunteers for a turn.

Teacher: How would you like to experiment with this today?

While I often ask this as a lesson starts, I do so today particularly to create another opportunity for decision-making in this lesson, especially because I suspect that the "had to"–a verbal representation of lack of choice–is at least a contributing factor to the headaches. Offering multiple-choice opportunities throughout the lesson highlights freedom to choose.

Student: I don't know…I think the transcription is going much better, and the headaches are milder than they were… (*she pauses, looking surprised*) Wow, just thinking about going to work, I notice that I started to tighten.

Teacher: Yes, great that you noticed that. We could start with that—just using the Alexander Technique to think about work…does that sound useful?

Offering another moment of choice.

Student: Yeah, I should try that (*starts*)…argh, I don't even like to think about it.

I note the "should" and choose not to mention it yet.

Teacher: Tell me about your job—what is it? How did you get it? Do you like it?

Student: It's the perfect job for me if I have to have a job! I am a receptionist for a law firm; they let me go to auditions during the day if I need to. It pays better than most of the jobs I can get, and I don't have to wait tables.

Teacher: I have been hearing a lot of "have to" and "should" language when you talk about your work.

> *The whole group has been included all along; at this moment, I bring them more directly into the discussion.*

One of the things we have talked about is that the Alexander Technique can be a barometer for constructive thinking. "Shoulds" and "have tos" belong to the category of nonconstructive thinking. We generally tighten between head and spine when we are "shoulding" ourselves.

Student: But I do have to go to work!

Teacher: Odd as it sounds to hear it, you don't have to go. You might lose your job if you don't go, and that will have consequences for you, but you don't have to.

Student: But then I couldn't pay the rent…

Teacher: Could you get another job?

Student: I have had other jobs and this is the one that works the best.

Teacher: It sounds to me like you want this job.

Student: Maybe…probably.

Teacher: You obviously don't like everything about it; you don't have to like something to want it.

> *I watch Student to see if this thought is easing the tightening between head and spine, and it is.*

I have an idea. Why don't we create a doorway to be the door to the building you work in, then you could practice walking in the building knowing you want to be there and see what happens?

> *Waiting for assent, another choice moment.*

Student: Okay.

Members of the class bring a few chairs to one part of the room to create a doorway. I offer quick turns to everyone as they rearrange the room.

Student, asking herself to coordinate, approaches the door and suddenly stops, tightening between head and spine, looking angry.

Student: I don't want to...

Teacher: That's clear. What happened just then?

Student: I am so angry. I want to be able to be an actor without having to have a day job. I don't want to be a receptionist. I am so angry that I can't just be an artist!

On that last sentence, Student makes a large arm gesture and I note, without commenting, that the gesture is beautifully coordinated.

Teacher: Wow, I so agree. It is so hard to be an artist and hold a day job and not have as much time or energy for what you care about most.

I teach a lot of artists and resonate with Student's plight, choosing to reveal that I share the anger this artist has expressed. I am metaphorically walking with the emotional response, partially in empathy, but also assuring that the strong emotion is welcome in the room, natural, and safe. I also look around the room to see if any members of the group are concerned; in this case, everyone has experienced the safety of emotional reactions in their Alexander Technique classes, so I don't need to offer any additional information. I look around the room, knowing there are other artists in the class.

Does anyone else recognize this issue?

A few heads nod. Someone tells a story about what he says to himself when he is at work and starts to feel angry or sad about it.

Do you have any other options for work right now?

Student: Not really.

Teacher: Okay...I have an offer. Would it work for you to consider that the truth about you is that you want to go to this job for right now, knowing it is the best job *right now* for supporting your acting?

Offering another choice.

Student: That is the truth. Let's see what happens.

We experiment multiple times with walking to the door and reaching for the doorknob. With the reaching for the handle, we review some of the arm action information from the week before. With each experiment, Student is able to sustain her coordination a little longer. Eventually she is able to go inside the "doorway." It takes a lot of willpower, which is why I started decision-making practice early in the lesson. Because the emotional component is strong, I want to add more challenge to the learning.

Teacher: Let's get this a little more real, shall we?

Waiting for assent.

Is everyone willing to pretend we are all downtown walking past this building?

This turn is taking a longer time than most, while traveling some pretty serious territory. I am looking for a way to take Student's learning one step further while also involving the group. The topics covered in the lesson are applicable to everyone. A component I hope will emerge is enjoyment in the success of the new plan, which would probably increase the likelihood that Student will be able to carry it through on her own later.

(*to Student*) Would that be okay?

Waiting again for assent; Student nods her head.

As we are all walking, you can decide anytime you want to go in our imaginary door. If you start to go in and notice that you start to tighten, you can just go around the block again.

Everyone in the room joins in—we are pretending to walk around the block in Seattle where she works. I am doing quick walking turns with everyone, including Student. While I watch, Student has several aborted entries, deciding to walk around the block rather than go inside. Several times, however, she uses the Alexander

Technique to help her walk through a door she wants to go through.
Seeing success, I want to add another element.

Is it okay if I invite everyone who might want to practice walking
through a doorway that is challenging to them to join you?

The quick walking turns continue for a few minutes; several people
experiment with going through the doorway. This is an example of
a moment in which students can have privacy within the group. No
one is asked to explain the content of their chosen challenge. It is a
deep play game–invented for this particular class at this moment in
time. Smiles and laughter appear as people play with choices in the
doorway–there are some traffic jams, as well as squeals and groans
as people confront their personal challenges. One person finally runs
through the doorway–in great coordination–and everyone cheers.
Spontaneously they all start running through the doorway.

Amazing! (*bringing this section of the class to a close*) And isn't it true that
on the other side of a challenge, there is often joy?! (*checking in with*
Student) Do you have what you need to continue the experiment?

Student: Yes, I am curious to go to work tomorrow.

Teacher: Does anyone else have any comments or needs about this
question?

It is especially important to ask this question after a turn like this.
It is possible that someone else in the room has a similar question,
or that this turn brought up something they'd like to follow up with.

Turn Three

One week later, at the beginning of class after the opening social
amenities.

Teacher: Does anyone have any reports, questions, or comments since
last time?

Student: I did the whole doorway thing the next day. It is a good thing
I went downtown a little early. I went around the block about five
times before I got in that door.

She is smiling and coordinating beautifully.

And the day was a whole lot better. I knew I was there because I wanted to be—if I started to think anytime during the day, "I don't want to be here," I remembered the walk around the building, and was able to use the Alexander Technique to do whatever I was doing. The headaches didn't happen.

Teacher: Fabulous work. And the lack of the headache will help your acting career, too. Did anyone else experiment with doorways this week?

And the class continues.

Student Two

He is a high school language arts teacher. He has gotten feedback that he looks stiff in front of his class, and he feels more exhausted at the end of a teaching day than he thinks he should.

Turn One

Teacher: Who would like a turn?

Student: I'd like to take a look at standing in front of my class.

Teacher: How shall we set up the room so that it looks a little more like a classroom?

> *Student and the rest of the group set up his classroom. I offer quick turns to people as they move the furniture.*

Do you want them (*indicating the rest of the group*) to be your students?

Student: That would be great.

Teacher: What grade?

Student: Tenth grade.

Teacher: Everyone who wants to can be a tenth-grade student. Just remember, you can be a reasonably behaved group of tenth graders.

> *Whenever adults take on the roles of children, I have found it helpful to mention this. Often, the first iteration of pretend classrooms can have everyone misbehaving wildly–I suspect they are doing everything they didn't do in tenth grade but wanted to!*

Okay, when you are ready, go ahead and greet your class.

Student goes to the front of the class, tightens his legs as he stands, and pulls his arms back as he inhales. Both of these actions have pulled him over backward, causing him to need to tighten the head–spine relationship and in a number of other places, including the jaw. As he exhales, he presses his arms down–because they are still pulled back, this pulls him even farther backward.

Student: Good morning, class!

He does look stiff because he is stiff and his voice is squeezed.

Teacher: Go ahead into what you might do next so I can see what happens.

He teaches for a little while. I see him start to give up much of the extra work he did at the beginning, but it looks like as soon as he senses the absence of the pull back of his arms, he pulls them back again.

Is there anything you are noticing about yourself as you teach in this imagined classroom? (*to the group*) Is there anything you are noticing?

Group: A few mention the overall pressure in his system; one comments on how far back the arms are.

Student: My arms are back, what do you mean?

Someone in the group demonstrates.

Teacher: Do you recognize that movement?

Student: I do. When I was student teaching, I had trouble taking charge of the class. My supervising teacher suggested that I plant my feet, and then make sure I was open to the class, and then relax.

As he says this, he moves just as when he started to teach. I also notice a slight change in him as he says "my supervisor"–he looks lighter and his voice gets a bit warmer.

Teacher: It looks like you enjoyed your supervising teacher.

Student: I did. I really struggled with discipline in the classroom those first weeks and she helped me figure out how to do it, and never made me feel badly about it.

I note his appreciation of nonjudgmental learning.

Teacher: I love that. What changed things for you?

Student: She told me about planting my feet and all that in the spring before when I was visiting her class, but what really changed it for me was how, when I came to student teach, she mentored me through every step of setting up my classroom, and how to lay out the rules and expectations for the class. She was pretty bossy about it! (*laughing*) I guess because she'd have to deal with class discipline if I didn't— but I am really glad she did it.

Teacher: She sounds great. Does she plant her feet and all that?

The word "bossy" jumps out from what he said. I wonder if he has some aversion to being in charge. I don't know and will keep wondering about it.

Student: (*pausing to imagine his supervising teacher moving; as he thinks of her, his coordination improves a bit*) No, she just moves fluidly around her room.

Teacher: So, it sounds like what I am going to name the "planting your feet" sequence isn't what actually helped you?

Student: (*getting it, a bit excited*) No...it wasn't.

He faces the room as if to start teaching again...and pauses.

Wow, when I consider starting without doing that sequence, I get really scared.

Teacher: What are you concerned with? Or about?

Student: I am afraid the students won't listen to me unless I show them I'm the boss.

Teacher: Okay...let's see if we can find a way to take care of your fear. You said earlier that your supervising teacher was a bit bossy with you, what did you mean by that? What did she do that made you call her bossy?

Student: She insisted that I do every step of her planning process, write it out in my own words, and do it in class. After the class, we would review what happened in class to see how I carried through with my intention, thought of alternatives, and then did the same thing again for the next day.

Teacher: That sounds a lot like what you said worked about classroom discipline—the clarity of the step-by-step process and the expectations. Let's start the class again and, this time, what if you start teaching this lovely tenth-grade class by first asking yourself to COORDINATE so that your head can move so that all of you can follow so that you can look around and see that you are safe; then asking yourself to COORDINATE so that your head can move so that all of you can follow so that you can invite your students to be with you while you are with them so that you can tell them what you are doing in class today?

> *I am using my hands to follow him as he changes as a "yes" to the new communication idea. After a few moments watching him teach, I pause.*

What do you think?

> *He is able to leave off all the complication of the "planting your feet" sequence rather easily.*

Student: It feels a lot better but I am not convinced it will work.

Teacher: That makes sense—you've been doing it the other way for a while. (*to the group*) Does anyone else have any feedback for him?

Group: "He looked more comfortable." "It was easier to listen to him."

Teacher: I have an idea. Since your concern was discipline, what if I ask this pretend class to be a little less cooperative, and we play with this again?

Student: Okay.

> *We have several rounds of this with the pretend tenth graders getting gradually more rowdy. Each time, he uses the plan above, and the rowdiness subsides and the class comes together.*

Group: "When you are so clear, it is hard to decide to be rowdy."

Teacher: It is an option you can explore with your real students this week. You can always go back to your previous plan if the new one doesn't work, and I think it will work well and potentially take care of you better. Any thoughts or questions?

Later in the class, I will hope to touch on elements of his earlier pattern—the leg tightening to "plant," the pullback of the arms mistakenly thinking that makes him "open," and the press down on the exhale—in activities with the whole group, or perhaps in one of the individual turns. This turn seems complete in the moment because he has a constructive replacement plan. Because he easily stopped doing the "planting your feet" sequence, I don't want to call direct attention to the old pattern again. A little indirect information about any of the component parts of his "planting" sequence will probably be helpful later.

Turn Two

One week later.

Student: I can't believe I have been doing all that other stuff for so long. The new plan worked fine because it wasn't all of that pushing myself around that was creating the discipline—it was the process my supervising teacher taught me. Classes were so much less stressful—I had no idea how much work I was putting into just standing there. I even got to laughing in one class—which somewhat mystified the students—because I was writing on the board a lot and every time I turned back around to face them, I started to do the old pattern. I changed to the new one right away. It happened so much that it got to be funny—I have no idea what the students thought, but they kept paying attention.

Another person in the group: I teach, too, and, after last week, I realized that I had a bit of a "get ready" routine, too. It was the word "bossy" that stuck with me. I realized that I didn't want to be "bossy," so I was doing this funny floppy heavy "relax" thing to signal that I wasn't the boss. And the kids often behave as if I am not the boss. Watching and listening to you last week, I realized that it is my job to be in charge, and if I used the plan you came up with, "ask myself to COORDINATE so that my head can move so that all of me can follow so that I can invite my students to be with me while I am with them so that I can guide the class," I didn't feel bossy yet was in more control of the room. So, thanks!

Teacher: Wonderful experiments! Anyone else have any reports or questions?

Student Three

This student introduced herself to me as a massage therapist who wanted to study with me because a friend—another massage therapist—told her that it really helped her mechanics in massage.

Turn One

Teacher: Does anyone have something they'd like to explore?

Student: My low back started to hurt again while I was massaging and I still can't figure out what is happening.

> *As she talks, I omniserve. In previous weeks, we have worked quite meticulously on the mechanics of many of her massage strokes, using the Alexander Technique at each change of stroke.*

Teacher: I am sorry to hear that…it had gone away for a while, hadn't it?

Student: Yes.

Teacher: Sounds like you have been doing some detective work about it…what have you found out so far?

> *I want to honor her work, and it will also expedite this lesson to hear her clues.*

Student: Not much, I kept reviewing what we did and asking myself to COORDINATE to do each thing and it didn't seem to be helping.

> *Noting the frustration, I wonder what has changed. Is she starting to try to recreate the feeling and not the process? Is one of the old ideas returning? She had had a strong pattern of tightening her legs to feel grounded–has that pattern reemerged?*

Teacher: Did you bring your massage table?

Student: Yes.

Teacher: Shall we set it up and see if we can get more clues?

Student: Let's do it.

The members of the class help rearrange the room and one calls out, "I'll be your client." Student starts the massage. As I omniserve, I see something new. As Student switches to a new stroke, her abdomen is pushing out. I continue to watch.

Teacher: I do see something. How would you describe breathing while you massage?

Student: I don't know what I used to do, but I just started yoga and most of what we are doing is working on breathing so I am thinking to ask to COORDINATE to take a nice low breath when I change strokes.

As she describes it, she does the abdomen pushing out pattern. I strongly suspect that some mistaken idea of what a low breath is has caused the return of the back pain.

Teacher: (*to the whole class*) Everyone, what do you imagine someone means when they say "breathe low"?

Everyone considers how to answer the question as Student answers immediately.

Student: What the yoga teacher said was to start filling in from the bottom, so to fill the bottom near the pelvis floor first, then a little above, and a little more above until you are full.

Teacher: Think about your anatomy...are the lungs in your low abdomen?

Student looks a little startled, because, as a massage therapist, she does know more anatomy than most people. It dawns on her that there is a mismatch between what the yoga teacher said and what she actually knows. To prevent her–I hope–from feeling bad about what she is starting to realize is a "mistake," I quickly continue.

A lot of people talk about "low breathing." I know what they are asking for, but the way they ask for it sometimes causes trouble.

A whole group discussion of how breathing works ensues, with visual aids, then the group experiments with humming. Many quick turns on various aspects of breathing punctuate the didactic information.

Okay, let's take this back to the massage. It could be quite skillful to take a conscious breath each time you switch strokes. If you select a plan that cooperates with the design of breathing, let's see what happens.

> *I see Student using the Alexander Technique to carry out the new plan for breathing, occasionally using my hands to communicate, following her as she tries out the new plan.*

Student: Yeah, that seems to have cleared things up.

Teacher: Anyone else have any questions about breathing, or is there something else you would like to explore?

Turns Make Theory Practice

Years ago, when someone asked my five-year-old daughter what the Alexander Technique is, she said, "It just means you don't have to squish up your neck all the time." I thought, yes, that is pretty much it. Simple. Marj frequently said to us, "It's just too simple for you."

What I sometimes say is, "The Alexander Technique is pretty simple. What sometimes gets complicated is what we are doing to ourselves." It is through the endless variety within turns that this simple tool gets its practical "legs." Chapter 30, "Tips for Turns," follows up on a few of those variations.

Chapter 22

TEACHING GROUPS

The turns described in the previous chapter transpired within group classes. When I visit Alexander Technique training schools, I remind them on the first day that I learned the Alexander Technique solely in a group setting, and didn't know that anyone even took private lessons until after I was already teaching. Since everything I learned about the Alexander Technique and teaching it happened in groups, I have full confidence that group teaching is effective. While I approach teaching pretty much the same no matter how many people are in the room, the following discussion relates the skills in previous chapters specifically to group teaching.

Adult Group Learning

Most of us learned in groups as children. While there are some commonalities between children's group learning and adult learning, there are also significant differences that affect how you set up a group. Adult education specialist Jean Illsley Clarke defines the characteristics of an effective leader of an adult group:

> Warmth, particularly noting goodwill and trust in people
>
> Indirectness, being able to help people discover learning
>
> Organized, via steps and resources for specific learning goals
>
> Enthusiastic about subject and about learners.
>
> (Clarke 1998, pp. 14–15)

She notes that what gets in some people's way is thinking of leading the group as they experienced their childhood education—pedagogy. Her three-step description of pedagogy is to say what you are going to teach, teach it, then say what you taught. "However, as people mature, [adults] want to become more and more in charge of their own learning and to have leaders who use androgogy" which is "based on the assumption that both the leader and the learners are capable of making quality contributions and of reaching competent conclusions" (Clarke 1998, p.42) As an alternative to the three steps of pedagogy, she offers:

The parallel adage for teaching mature people is:

- First you and they set the goals.

- Then you tell them briefly what you have to offer and how it relates to their goals.

- Next you provide the opportunity for them to explore, to experience, and to share what they have to offer.

- Finally you ask them what they have learned.

(Clarke 1998, p.42)

Regarding Clarke's characteristics of an effective adult group leader, I assume that anyone caring enough about teaching the Alexander Technique to read this book has the characteristics of warmth and enthusiasm. I discuss the organizational aspects in Chapter 20.

With the Alexander Technique, we define our work as indirect because we focus on the means-whereby to an end rather than the end itself. What Clarke defines as "indirect" is similar in that the teacher is supplying the means by which the student can learn. She says, "it means leading learning experiences in such a way that allows people to discover information and concepts for themselves" (Clarke 1998, p.43). Clarke refers to Knowles in her suggestions on this topic:

Knowles suggests, among other things, that facilitators of adult learning provide indirectness by:

- Offering mutual negotiation of objectives.

- Giving adults chances to learn from each other.

- Using experiential (doing) as well as transmitting (telling and showing) techniques.

- Providing an informal, respectful, collaborative climate.

(Clarke 1998, p.44)

The flow of an adult group class comes from the willingness to be a leader who is a co-collaborator with the participants in the learning community. One who is in action, ready to provide resources as needed, to devise learning events as needed, and to witness learning.

Following are discussions on common questions I receive about group teaching.

Individual and Whole-Group Balance

You are teaching everyone always. Moderating the balance of the class so that individuals' questions are addressed and everyone fully participates is primarily the teacher's responsibility. An element that facilitates your ability to moderate the flow of the group is teaching the students what their responsibilities are. I ask my students to...

- Arrive with something they want to do.

- Ask questions at any time, particularly right when they have them.

- Feel free to move as they need, and to do the same thing that is happening in an individual lesson whenever they want.

- Know that if I invite everyone to do something, they may choose to watch instead.

- Exercise freedom of choice in question answering, that is, "You can tell me something," "You can say 'I don't know,'" "You can say 'I don't want to tell you.'"

- Tell me if they would prefer not to have touch as a component of the teaching process.

My introductory class proffers these "jobs" for the student in a largely informal way. As I teach the class based on these assumptions, I find that students take on their jobs easily, perhaps occasionally needing a renewal.

I function something like a tour guide as I teach the turns, so everyone knows where we are in the sequence of wanting–recognizing–deciding–gathering information–creating a plan–inviting yourself to action. I may not mention every step, yet I do every step every time, choosing to call attention to aspects of the process as necessary for the group. When teaching an individual within the group, you are reinforcing everyone's learning.

If the students arrive already knowing what they'd like to explore or what questions they have, that is a timesaver. It also means they know everyone else has a request, too; their awareness of the community helps me balance the time.

I omniserve throughout; quizzical looks may prompt a choice to offer more information verbally, or asking, "Do you have a question?" Almost always at the end of a lesson, I ask, "Do you have any comments?" "Do you have any questions?" Even if people don't directly answer me at that point, I know that simply putting the question in the air helps everyone review what just happened.

What may emerge from end-of-lesson questions reveals the richness of group learning: people may be reminded of something they want to explore, may discover an application of the Alexander Technique they never thought of, or may offer expertise from their own area(s). Frequently, an individual lesson becomes a whole-group exploration of an activity or a question.

You are always teaching the whole group. I intend to give participants some time dedicated to their particular want or question. Somewhat informally and by no means rigidly, I think in terms of two to three individual turns, then an activity with the group. If one of the individual lessons becomes something the whole group explores, then that is the "group" moment.

Time management is important, and I take it seriously in my planning. I have accepted that part of my contract with the group is to begin and end on time. Adults have a lot of competing commitments; my timeliness respects their needs. My hope always is to respond to what everyone has come to learn within the time we have. As a young teacher, if I occasionally felt panicky about getting around to everyone, I would remember one of Marj's workshops with more than 50 people. I was deeply affected watching Marj teach a turn that took a long time. It took a long time

> **TEACHING STORY**
> When Cathy was teaching Diego, giving him some help with his eyes, I noticed a change in the area of his cheekbones which spread towards his ears. Then I noticed a change in myself! The area around my ears opened up and then my perception of the sounds and sights in the room changed and became more pleasurable. Especially the view out the window. It was as if the sun had just come out. My shift came from thinking about an outward observation. Next, we looked at the pictures of the muscles of the head in an anatomy book. I was sure I saw the muscles around my ears that had shifted. Amazing way to learn.

because it needed to take a long time. As a novice teacher, what I learned was "Each lesson takes the time it takes." While I may have an overall time management framework, it is imperative to value the needs of the current circumstances.

More important than the intention to do two or three lessons and then a group activity is diligent attention to teaching everyone all the time. Questions I ask are to everyone. Everyone does not need to have an individual turn to learn or enjoy the class. When I read student journals from the university, I frequently find out that a "breakthrough" someone has in understanding the Alexander Technique came from watching someone else's lesson. If anyone seems to be outside the group, I include them visually and with my gestures as I teach.

Often, I don't need to do anything special visibly for the individual and whole-group balance—it flows seamlessly. Consistent practice helps, as does the group's understanding of their role in the process.

Privacy in a Group

One of the group's responsibilities, that they know they don't need to answer any question they don't want to answer, is a jointly carried responsibility. I keep my word. Sometimes, I need to remind other members in the group of our shared agreement. If a moment in class seems to need privacy, I sometimes have a mini-very-quiet conversation to gather information and/or offer support as I also renew their freedom to choose. I may slightly turn my back to the rest of the group when I do this, to create a sort of privacy shield. On rare occasions, the conversation may move to another space, or we may take a break so the group is busy while we finish talking.

Omniserving in a Group Class

My omniservation skills were initially developed for theatre. Before I had any concern whatsoever about head–spine relationships, I was in countless acting classes, deciphering what worked and what didn't, what revealed, what concealed. Manuel Duque, my Meisner teacher at Penn State, taught us not only to find our own sense of truth, but also to recognize it in others.

Another of my acting professors at Penn State, Kelly Yeaton, used mirror exercises in actor training, and even directed a show with a full mirror cast. In graduate school at Washington University in St. Louis, I wrote and directed a mirror play for two actresses—both of whom could play both roles. We never knew who would start the play—it emerged from what happened as they began to mirror each other. As a director and acting teacher, mirroring partner games are one of my consistent tools, particularly when creating an embodied relationship between characters who have a long history.

Usually, in doing a mirror exercise, two people stand opposite each other. In the beginning version, one person is designated the leader, and the other is the follower. My instruction, somewhat modified from what I was taught, is to look at the other person with your general focus primarily in the head to sternum area—a kind of circle around the head. The leader moves, and the follower follows as close to simultaneously as possible. Periodically, the teacher/director says, "switch," and seamlessly the leader becomes the follower and vice versa. Eventually, you can do leaderless mirrors, opposite mirrors, and mirrors with more than two people. Many variations are possible.

The mirrors are active practice in whole-self communication, including the "bubble around the body," and a huge exercise in omniservation. Mirrors also teach to omniserve "whole" rather than to track all the parts directly; this kind of omniservation is easier and less intrusive for the student. As a theatre artist, I have been trained continually to omniserve, to take in the whole picture with the intention of receiving/being with my partner. My job in a play is to respond to my onstage partners while inviting the audience into our story. What an actor needs onstage is exactly what an Alexander Technique group teacher needs.

If theatre isn't in your background, how do you develop the skill? One activity is to watch people walking down the street and play with mirroring them—subtly, subtly—you don't want them to know you are omniserving them. Just as you wouldn't want your student to feel "scrutinized," you don't want these "civilians" to know you are gathering details about how they are moving. In Alexander Technique language, this is a practice of Frank Pierce Jones's "integrated field of attention" (Jones 1997, p.9).

Rhythm/Tempo

The rhythm and tempo of a class need to vary. What I mean by "rhythm" is the pattern of lesson to lesson; what I mean by "tempo" is the speed of that rhythm. As with music, if tempo or rhythm is relentlessly predictable, people tend to stop listening (except perhaps on a dance floor). They are lulled into a passive state. In *Tips: Ideas for Actors*, Jon Jory says, "Rhythm has to vary more often than any but the very best of us realize. After three or four sentences, the rhythm begins to lull the auditor rather than grab them. Thinking about rhythm needs to be part of your creative process. Talk is jazz" (Jory 2000, p.57).

Coordinating to teach at any needed tempo is a skill worth developing, so we can respond to our students at the pace they need. We all individually have a preferred tempo/rhythm. In several communication classes I have taught for Alexander Technique teachers, we discovered some people need practice in continuing to coordinate at a tempo/rhythm that is outside their own preferences.

As a founding faculty member for the Performance School, my particular specialty was teaching an Alexander Technique-infused acting class, with the intention of teaching communication skills as well as serving the performers who were in the class. On the very first day, I started my well-planned class and was shocked when no more than ten minutes into the class, everyone was angry with me. That had never happened to me before; I was teaching material I had taught many times successfully. We worked through the situation and in essence restarted the class. Afterward, I reviewed what had happened to see how I could improve. When I got to the circumstance question, "What time is it?" I was pretty sure I knew what had happened. The class before mine was a tai chi class. My students had been moving very, very, very slowly for an hour before I arrived. Acting classes generally move at a fairly fast pace, and I came in teaching at that pace. I surmised that it was the drastic shift in rhythm/tempo pace that caused the communication difficulty. The next class, I slowed down my own pace before walking in. I started to speak to them at a slow tempo...and very gradually sped up. It worked. I needed to do this every week.

The way I described my process—"I slowed down my own pace"—is something I learned as an actor. To create a character other than ourselves, actors need to know how we respond to situations, including tempo/rhythm, and learn how to mink and thove in the tempo/rhythm of the character.

To give you an idea of the detailed study possible, here is the beginning of an exercise from Michael Chekhov:

> Create an improvisation preferably with a group, distinguishing between the outer and inner Tempos. For example, choose a scene in an operating room... The inner Tempo is extremely fast. All movements and short cues on the contrary, are cautious, controlled and reserved. The outer Tempo is slow. (Chekhov 1991, p.144)

He goes on to offer many variations of improvisation, mixing and matching inner and outer tempo in many ways.

Another example, related to musical performance, might help clarify what I am talking about. A musician was readying himself to play a scherzo by calming himself down. He got himself thinking slowly, then tried to play something very fast. The incongruity caused him to tighten between head and spine. The concern he had brought to his lesson was that he was always behind the tempo he wanted. When I coached him to think in the tempo he wanted—with the excitation of the scherzo—the tightening between his head and spine disappeared. He was now thinking and playing matching tempos.

We might need to mismatch rather than match the speed of our students. In the Performance School class described above, my plan began by matching and then gradually speeding everyone up. One of my students frequently got stuck in learning. She stayed in a fairly deliberate rhythmic pattern—it could be fast or slow, but was always similarly rhythmic. When I varied my own rhythms rather than matching her, she could learn more easily.

Small Groups within the Large Group

Breaking into smaller groups within a large group workshop is a useful change of pace. In Chapter 17, I mentioned the small groups that Marj used to help build our communication skills. Key to their success is giving them a specific task to accomplish in a specified period of time. Other possibilities for small-group assignments could include asking each group to analyze a particular movement; giving each group a paragraph from something you'd like everyone to read, then asking the group to come up with a skit that demonstrates the paragraph; or asking each group to talk about what they learned from a lesson everyone just watched. The possibilities are limitless. Small groups are valuable because they add variety to the structure, make it easier for reticent people to talk, and are another way for adults to actively participate in their own learning.

If you have experienced students, or students who are learning to teach the Alexander Technique, it is a good opportunity to put them "in charge" of a small group. Their job is to guide the group so that it stays on the given task.

As a playful ending to some of my large groups, I create play stations for people to experiment with different tasks related to the Alexander Technique. For example, if I have a group of 30, I might ask them to form five groups of six people. My five play stations might be: (1) Spine puzzle—all the vertebrae are separated, and the task is to put them together as a puzzle; (2) Hula hoops; (3) Tip the Waiter game— to experiment with physics and geometry in omniservation by trying to stack a toy waiter's tray with wooden "food" without knocking him over (as well as using the Alexander Technique to move your hands); (4) Sudoku; (5) Blowing bubbles. Everyone might get seven minutes at each station to play with using the Alexander Technique for the given tasks. Everyone gets a lot of Alexander Technique practice in a dense period of time.

Variety Is the Spice of Teaching

My own preference in learning is to be active. This is not everyone's preference. What is most important for me in teaching is knowing that each of us has our own preferences. Knowles's discussion of individual differences acknowledges the plethora of approaches and incomplete research "but the key point is clear: Individuals differ in their approaches, strategies, and preferences during learning activities" (Knowles *et al.* 2005, p.216). He notes, and this is my point, too, that simply knowing that we all learn differently already begins to change how you approach teaching.

The styles most are familiar with are audio, visual, or kinetic learners. Whether someone considers themselves an introvert or an extrovert, or a big-picture or little-picture learner are also factors. Carol Dweck's research in mindsets adds another element to consider: whether someone has a fixed idea of themselves or a growth mindset, "based on the belief that your basic qualities are things you can cultivate through your efforts" (Dweck 2006, p.7). In researching play for this book, I discovered a classification of people by preferred play styles: the joker, the kinesthetic, the explorer, the competitor, the director, the collector, the artist/creator, and the storyteller (Brown 2009, pp.66–70).

Knowing what you prefer is important so that you don't impose your preference on everyone. This also enables you to offer things you yourself might not need as a learner, because you know someone might need it.

I never used to write things down on a chalkboard, or hand out much written material—this never occurred to me because it wasn't part of how I learned. Now I do, and I can see that it helps some people. When I experience that some way I am communicating does not seem to be effective, I continue listening, watching, and experimenting with other ways of saying or doing the same thing—I start varying my presentation. When in doubt, change what you are doing somehow!

Spice it up:

- Switch to a game.

- If you've been working slowly on detail, do some quick turns.

- Bring out a reference.

- Tell a pertinent story.

- Give the group a specific task on the next turn.

- Divide into small groups with specific tasks.

- Suggest everyone get up and take a walk.

- Offer a writing or drawing task.

- If the group has been loud, offer a quiet task.

- If the group has been quiet, offer a task that uses sound.

- Have an anatomy exploration related to a particular lesson.

- Play a game that is really just for fun.

- Stand in a different part of the room.

- Ask the group to sit in a different part of the room (literally seeing the work from a different direction).

- Go outside.

- Have a tea break.

- Pick an Alexander Technique or related reading and ask each person to read one sentence.

Remember, Above All...

From the smallest group of the private lesson to the largest groups, you are teaching everyone, all of the time.

Chapter 23

TEACHING AN INTRODUCTION

The introductory class is perhaps the one most of us will end up teaching most often. Because it has a specific purpose, one that has common elements—whether for 1 person or 100 people—I have planned many versions of this gateway experience. One day, my host at the University of Idaho scheduled me for eight introductions in one day; when I realized he was going to be at all of them, I did my best to make them all a little bit different. At another university, they simply told everyone I would be in a room all day, so people kept wandering in and out as their class schedules permitted. I needed to cycle new versions of the introduction every half hour or so—highlighting new elements for people who were already in class while orienting any new arrivals.

Spending considerable time on what you want to include in your introduction and actually writing, or at least outlining, many versions is a recommended task. *My goal in teaching an introduction to the Alexander Technique is to teach in such a way that if this person never had a lesson again, they would be able to continue experimenting with the process on their own. At the same time, I intend to give them the information they need to see if the Alexander Technique matches what they want for themselves.* What I hope they remember is the nonjudgmental playful learning environment, freedom of choice, and that the head–spine relationship serves as a coordination barometer we have the ability to consciously cooperate with in service of what we want to do. Throughout an introduction, these goals deeply inform my teaching decisions. As I hear how students respond, I answer in a frame that continually returns to these emphases.

Introductory Class Elements

Although my introductions take many forms, they generally include:

- Finding out what brought people to the studio and what they already know about the Alexander Technique or expect the Alexander Technique to do for them.

- Explaining that because the Alexander Technique is about how you do what you do, you need a "what to do."

- Offering at least one, usually several, practical activities that illustrate how the head–spine relationship affects overall coordination.

- Guiding participants through the AT Progression to do something before I use my hands in the teaching process.

- Explaining how I could use my hands as part of the teaching/communication process and asking permission to use touch.

- Applying the Alexander Technique to something they care about, something related to why they came, using any teaching tools that seem appropriate. (*Note:* this is an important aspect of helping them decide whether the Alexander Technique might be useful to them in their lives—applying it to something they care about.)

- Teaching them to use an external cue (such as, "When you reach for a cup, you could…") to rehearse the new process.

- Encouraging them to experiment with the new ideas.

- Giving them information about what continued study offers and letting them know how to continue if they want to.

What I usually refer to directly or indirectly as the lesson progresses:

- How our senses work.

- How we think we are designed may affect our coordination (bringing in anatomical information as necessary, though I prefer to keep this minimal in the first class).

- That saying "yes" to the new idea is what replaces the older idea (reiterating that we do perfectly what we know how to do based on the information we have).

- Offering a colorful postcard with the essential Alexander Technique "ask" on it to give them at the close of the introduction.

What I might need to do:

- Give my background, my Alexander Technique story.

- Credential myself if I offer ideas contrary to their previous learning.

- In rare instances, if there is a significant medical issue, I may want to request information from their health-care professionals.

Written versions of my current introduction exist in a variety of publications (including Madden and Juhl 2017, "Report on a Five-Day Introductory Class for the University of Washington School of Drama," pp.262–276). Following is a version that highlights my use of the invented verb.

An Introduction Using an *Invented Word*

From a talk I gave at the 2011 Alexander Technique Congress in Lugano for teachers about the element of play in teaching. It was originally published as part of the Congress Papers (Madden 2012, pp.85–88).

"Welcome to this introduction to the Alexander Technique. I am delighted to be able to offer you some information about this practical tool that you can use in your daily and professional lives.

To begin, we need to pick something to do. The Alexander Technique is about 'how' you do what you do rather than about what you do. To teach a 'how' we need a 'what.' I am going to suggest that we use picking something up off the floor near our chairs as our 'what' for this introduction. As we experiment, just know that picking this object up simply represents anything we might do in our lives—from sitting and breathing to making a business presentation to doing the dishes to writing computer code to singing a song." (*Note:* My intention is to set up a deep play situation in which the group can discover that the dynamic relationship between head and spine is a key factor in vertebrate coordination, essentially recreating in a condensed form F.M. Alexander's original discovery.)

"Now, please go ahead and pick the object up as you usually would."

I look around the room and note, "Great—that worked, everyone was able to pick up their objects."

"Now, it is often easiest to understand an important element in vertebrate coordination if we start with what I call a little 'reverse' Alexander. Would you please scrunch just a tiny bit (I demonstrate) in the relationship between your head and your spine and then pick the object up again?" (I also demonstrate this.) (As everyone does this, there are usually some groans, some little gasps of surprise.)

"You all kindly scrunched up between head and spine in response to my request, did anything else change in you?"

Typical responses to my question include:

- It was heavier than before (physical).

- It hurt (physical).

- My range of movement decreased (physical).

- I forgot what you wanted us to do (thought).

- I didn't want to do it anymore (thought/emotion).

- I was less aware of my surroundings (sensory).

Not every group reports a full range of responses—that is, some groups may only report physical shifts and others mostly thought or emotion shifts. At this point, I will usually say something like: "People report many different changes when they introduce what I am going to call an interference in the relationship between the head and spine— sometimes they notice a change in how they move, sometimes they hear better or colors seem brighter, sometimes their mood changes or they notice they are thinking more clearly."

If the group does not report a particular kind of response, then I often tell a story from another group's experience that includes an aspect that has not been mentioned. It is important in the introduction at least to allude to all aspects of self because I am introducing (without introducing the jargon) psychophysical unity.

Next, I suggest: "For the next experiment, please start out scrunching between head and spine as you pick the object up and partway through picking it up change your mind and stop the extra scrunching."

Generally, everyone is able to do this and I can say, "I have shelves of books on this topic, but what you essentially did in this experiment was to use the Alexander Technique. There was an interference in the relationship between your head and spine in movement that affected the quality of what you were doing and you were able to improve the quality of your task as you were doing it simply by choosing to restore the coordination of your head and spine."

It is at this point that I introduce the *invented word*—the word is defined as the moment of restoring the relationship between head and spine, cooperating with the design of human coordination. (I like to mention some time during the introduction that you do not need to have something going "wrong" to use the Alexander Technique, noting that most of the time when I use the Alexander Technique it is not to restore coordination, but to invite myself to cooperate with my design because I care about the quality of what I am about to do.)

"We need a word to represent this moment of choice. In my experience, it works best to invent a word for this process. Any word that we already know carries our past meanings with it. If we want to embrace learning something new, it works best to have a new word, one that has no previous associations with it, one that we create meaning for by our discoveries in class."

At this point, I often introduce another model to describe the invented word in another way. (Explaining it in multiple ways is helpful since people learn in so many different ways.)

"Here is another representation of the Alexander Technique. Please put one finger up to represent your body (I do this, too) and use the other hand to create a very large head for the body." (I think it is important to acknowledge that the proportions are wrong.)

"The design of the head–spine relationship in human coordination is for the head to move freely in relationship to the spine so that we can, for instance, walk down the street." As I say this, I move my "head-hand" in multiple directions (up down right left) on top of the "finger-body" as I make my little human model walk down an imaginary street. Then, I explain that when we interfere with our coordination, the head is pulled towards the spine and ask everyone to push their "head-hand" towards the "finger-body" and ask them to walk this model down the imaginary street, noting that now the little human model's walk is less efficient/less comfortable. Then, just as in the first demonstration when they were picking things up, I ask them to restore the head–spine relationship of this hand/finger model.

It is at this moment that I say, "We need a word to represent this moment in the process. As I said earlier, it seems to be most efficient and effective to invent a word. Does anyone have any suggestions for our invented word?" (I can offer suggestions, and it is always fun when a group finds their own suggestion.) It is important that the made-up word does not evoke any particular sensations/images. Everyone in the group needs to be content with the choice. It can be a real word that does not mean anything about head and spine (for instance, one group chose the scientific name for a comb-headed jellyfish) or it can be just a group of sounds that the group likes—for instance, "zing-ha."

Often, in an introductory class, I will ask the class to repeat the earlier experiment—to start out scrunching between head and spine and then, when they decide to "unscrunch," to say the invented word out loud as they make the decision. Following that, I often begin teaching individual lessons within the group, using the invented word.

By introducing the invented word through experiences that the group shares, we develop meaning together. Multiple senses are involved. We move. We hear both my words and the students' comments/questions. Vision is involved as I demonstrate and as they watch each other. Depending on the choice of task, touch, texture, temperature, taste, and smell may be involved. With an opening round of teaching that uses the invented word, we deepen our experience of its meaning. To a certain extent, an invented word gives the teacher more control in defining the Alexander Technique.

Because the intent in the Congress paper was to explain how I use the invented word, my description of the class ends here. What usually follows are individual turns within the group (or with an individual if a private lesson), during which I continue to emphasize my primary goals: to create a playful learning environment, while demonstrating that learning to consciously cooperate with our designed head–spine relationship improves our effectiveness and our pleasure in our daily and professional tasks.

Creating Your Own Introduction

Specifying what you intend to teach, then creating steps toward that goal are the first steps in planning. For a perspective on the organizational aspect of planning, I offer a non-Alexander Technique topic as a starting point.

What if I am teaching a class in clowning and the goal of my class is to teach people to make a rose out of ribbon? I am teaching this as a skill to emphasize that clowns offer gifts to people.

What is my objective? To teach people how to make a rose out of ribbon.

What do I need for this? Enough ribbon for everyone to have a piece at least a yard long. Scissors would also be handy.

What are the steps in making a rose out of a ribbon?

1. Fold the ribbon in half, making a diagonal crease at the center.

2. Hold the ribbon in your left hand, with the bottom side of the folded ribbon perpendicular to the floor and the top side of the folded ribbon parallel to the floor, on the right side.

3. Take the right side of the ribbon and fold it under the left side of the ribbon. Now the horizontal piece of the ribbon has changed to the left side.

4. Take the ribbon that is perpendicular to the floor and fold it upward.

5. Continue folding whichever ribbon is on top under the lower ribbon, creating a square shape, until you have used most of the ribbon.

6. You now have a square of folded ribbon.

7. Hold the square in your left hand, and put your third finger lightly under the pile to hold it in place.

8. Put the ribbon strand that is above the bottom of the pile between your second and third fingers.

9. Keeping your third finger under the pile, take the upper ribbon in your right hand and lightly pull it toward the floor.

10. Watch the rose emerge.

In the AT Progression terms, the numbered list is the gathering of information that is necessary to make a rose out of ribbon; in Clarke's terms, it is the actions and resources needed for the class.

> As I continue planning for the class, I ask myself, "How might I create the conditions in which people would want to learn to make a rose?"

Before Class

I do the preparatory work to ready myself to teach, particularly renewing my desire to teach clowns the idea of offering a gift to people literally and figuratively. In AT Progression terms, this is Wanting, Recognizing, Deciding for myself as a teacher; in Clark's terms, I am in steps one and two, recognizing my values and my overall desire. I would also have ribbon and scissors on hand.

Options for the Beginning of Class

As people arrive, I could be making roses and giving them to people as I finish them. Or, I could be talking to them about something else, incidentally making the rose, then surprise them as the rose emerges. I could say, "I've learned a trick, would anyone else like to learn it?"

In this case, I am drawing out desire in the group—they have come for a clown class (and I did learn how to do this in a clown class), so desire for the particular task cannot be taken for granted. From the AT Progression, this is the wanting step for the participants; in the Clarke model, this would be another aspect of step 2 of the plan.

Options for the Middle of Class

(One of the many ways I could imagine doing this.)

First, I demonstrate making the rose again, this time saying what I am doing as I am doing it. (*Note*: I select this as the first step based on what happened the last time I taught a group to do this, so this step is based on my evaluation of the last time I taught rose making—level 6 of Clarke.)

Next, I pass out the ribbon and talk everyone, step by step, through the process. After each step, I look around to see if everyone is with me.

When I reach step 5, the "continue" step, I ask everyone to stay with me for each ensuing fold (again, based on a Clarke level 6 evaluation of last time).

For steps 7, 8, and 9, I explain it, watch them, and ask them to check each other's hand placement.

At step 10, I do it first, then they do it. Then, I look around the room, see how many roses there are and how many not-quite roses.

Repeat the whole sequence, giving everyone new ribbon, perhaps pairing successful rose makers with the not quite rose makers. Repeat until (hopefully) everyone has succeeded.

In Alexander Technique terms, I am using the reasoned-out plan to do the action of making the rose; in Clarke's terms, it is the teaching of the class.

Options for the End of Class

Since the reason I was teaching how to make the rose was about gifting, I could set up a clown circle of some kind so that people could give the rose they made to someone else. In AT Progression terms, this is the next step in the carrying out of the plan, connecting it to the larger purpose, which relates to Clarke's values and the teaching of the class. If I ask the participants what they experienced in making and then gifting the roses, I will have contributed to the gathering information and to creating a plan stages for future clown events; in Clarke's terms, I will have done some evaluation of the process.

Creating Your Introductions

I thought to emphasize the plural in this heading because you want to have many versions. Once you have many approaches, you are never stymied by the question, "What do you teach?" You will find yourself able to do an introduction at literally a moment's notice. I sometimes joke that I could be tapped on my arm and turn around and do an Alexander Technique introduction, and, it is true—I once did one while waiting for the check-in counter to open at a Tokyo airport.

I created an example outside of the Alexander Technique to introduce thinking of the beginning, middle, and end of a class because I thought a process with a tangible result might make this discussion more clear. With an Alexander Technique introductory class, our goals are this specific and concrete, just not demonstrably visible.

I noted my goals earlier. What are your specific goals?

Questions and Ideas for Preparation
Before Class

- ✓ Chapters 19 and 20: "Preparing for Teaching" and "Planning for Teaching."

- ✓ What do you hope your students will know at the end of the class?

- ✓ Do you need any resources?

- ✓ Knowing what you want the outcome to be, what is the sequence of steps that could lead there? (You might need to think backward from the end result. If, for instance, one of the goals is for everyone leaving the class to feel empowered to experiment with the new ideas, what steps do you need to take on the way?)

Beginning of Class

- ✓ What learning environment do you want to create?

- ✓ What first activity supports the goals you have for the class?

Middle of Class

- ✓ What are the steps you have selected?

- ✓ How do you plan to teach individuals within the group?

- ✓ How do you plan to involve the group?

- ✓ What ideas do you have to support the goals you have? These are ideas you may or may not use, yet are ready to use: stories, information, games, activities, and so forth.

End of Class

- ✓ What ideas do you have for bringing the threads of information together?

✓ What message do you want to leave your introductory class with?

✓ Do you want to have a specific activity or game?

✓ Do you want to invite your students to talk about what they have learned?

✓ How do you want to let them know about continued study?

✓ Usually, I use this opportunity to emphasize freedom of choice again. Something like "Thank you for coming. If you have any questions, please feel free to contact me. I have information about continued study options I'll offer at the door—you can try this out and see what you think. I also have a registration sheet for a series of lessons on the desk if you are ready to sign up now."

The point of the planning is readiness. Sometimes, you have a terrific plan, and all the circumstances change so that you do something else. That is okay. In fact, if you don't have a specific plan, it is much harder to adapt to circumstances. That isn't only my experience; other teachers echo it as well.

I planned an introduction for engineers that was fairly detailed and careful since I knew they may not have thought that much about their own design, and that the possibility of self-care as a strategy in business communication might be on their "edge" of comfort. Before my presentation, we all watched a video presentation on the history of the company. When I began the Alexander Technique introduction, I said, "How well would those airplanes work if the head of the plane was scrunched into the body of the plane?" They looked a little surprised, yet answered immediately—"Not at all." My response was "We are kind of the same way. Fortunately, we can still work with some scrunch between head and spine, but it is at a cost to efficiency and comfort." That ended up being the entire introduction—they understood it immediately, so we skipped the rest of my planned introduction, jumping immediately into the middle section—practical experiments.

Having a detailed plan–that you may or may not use–is the key to spontaneity and improvisation.

Chapter 24

THE DROP-IN CLASS

This chapter moves from one of the most structured and prepared classes to one that is also much practiced but impossible to completely prepare for. While you know when and where it is, along with an idea of who may come, you know whom you are teaching only when they walk in the door. The ability to navigate the improvisatory progression of drop-in classes is a fundamental skill necessary in even the most structured classes.

Weekly drop-in classes are a staple of my teaching studio. Its flexible form provides a low-key, low-commitment path for people to start studying the Alexander Technique. It is also a way for people to study consistently. While I endeavor to begin and end on time for every class, punctuality is particularly important in the drop-in classes because people often "wedge" a class in between other commitments.

These are generally multilevel classes—from complete beginners all the way to other Alexander Technique teachers. Since classes and workshops with Marj were multilevel, this feature is familiar and one I value. What beginners have to offer all of us is the gift of discovering again what underpins this work. And beginners learn faster when they can see what is possible with the work in the presence of experienced students.

Drop-In Class Sequence

My preparation for the class is informal; I consciously consider myself along with my potential students' and my desires. My goal is to create the conditions in which those who have chosen to attend can learn what they want to learn. When I enter my teaching studio, my means is to invite my students to be with me while I am with them so that

I can invite them to use the Alexander Technique toward their goals. From there, the AT Progression guides our explorations.

Beginning

Of course, we say hello. We ask after each other's lives. We know why we are here, so the conversation moves easily to Alexander Technique. Wanting, Recognizing, Deciding flows naturally from this social time: "Anything you are particularly interested in today?" "What brought you here today?" "Do you have any questions?" It is rare in my studio for people to arrive without an answer to one of these questions, because they know I will ask them.

As I hear the wants, I am noting them, and potentially organizing them, possibly fashioning an opening activity that includes aspects of all or many of the wants. If, for instance, one person wants to type at the computer, one wants to look at a swimming motion, someone wants to garden, and another person plays a French horn, I recognize they all want to do something with their arms. Out of this, I might create an opening activity for all of us to do—one possible game might be "Elephant" (see "Games Digest"); or, I could ask everyone to pick an arm movement or exercise, and fashion quick turns not only with their own movement, but with everyone's chosen movements— building some information for the ensuing activities with arms.

I could offer a round of quick walks. Or, particularly if many people arrived, and it appears that time might be an issue, I'll just move into "turns," the Middle of the class.

> **TEACHING STORY**
>
> A student who played the French horn was getting a bit stuck with the way his arms moved around the horn. For a while, you used your hands to teach him as he played, but since his arm movements during French horn playing were necessarily within a limited range, you made up a little arm movement game and had everyone in the group join in. The game was to balance a small book on the fingertips of one hand, then to see what kinds of movements were possible throughout our arm (and the rest of us) while maintaining the balance of the book. We came up with ways to move the book in all kinds of directions with different amounts of bending and rotation in different joints of the arm. Eventually, we passed a single book from person to person and each of us improvised one segment of a collective "book dance" before handing it off to the next person. When the student went back to playing the horn, the difference was dramatic: much more arm–torso differentiation and appropriate movement throughout the arms.

Middle

In a drop-in class, individual turns among the group are the center of the action. Our explorations are all about gathering information, creating plans, and experimenting. With the AT Progression as our faithful guide, we get to work.

Turn after turn, studied rehearsed plans and deliberate practice are brought to bear, with invitations to the group to participate in as many ways as I can come up with. In this setting, many people have learned to experiment along with me; everyone asks questions. While it is primarily my job to be attentive to people who are new to the group, many of my experienced students are also attentive to newcomers.

What happens in these classes is wide-ranging. Because I don't know who will be there or what they will ask, they are improvisatory. In truth, all classes share this improvisatory quality because you never really know what will happen. This is just exceptionally true of drop-in classes.

I track my time; I intend for everyone who comes to have time to explore their particular question. Usually, this works. In stating this, however, I remember the day it seemed as if everyone who had ever studied with me in Seattle turned up for this one-hour class. Unusually, I needed to leave right on time to attend an event at my daughter's school. Forty-five minutes into the class, two people I had never seen before arrived wanting an introduction to the Alexander Technique. Needless to say, not everyone got a turn that day; unfortunately, those two new people didn't get much of an introduction either. I did my best.

Because I maintain that I am teaching everyone in the group all the time, whether they get an actual turn is not the whole point of the class. I took many classes and workshops in which I didn't have an individual turn; I always learned a lot. Sometimes, someone doesn't actually want a turn. At the time of writing, in fact, I have a student often in my weekly drop-in class who prefers to learn solely by watching.

End

In my drop-in classes, the end is often informal. Usually, I have been offering "take-away" ideas through the Middle part of class, so there is little need to summarize. If a game or activity begins the class, a reprise can be fun. I attempt—not always successfully—to be available to talk with people after class in case anyone has any additional questions.

The drop-in class is a place where anything can happen; my job is to use the AT Progression as my navigation guide no matter where our explorations take us.

Chapter 25

THE INTRODUCTORY SERIES

While I enjoy teaching mixed-level classes and workshops, an introductory series of classes offers the opportunity to tailor the content to the needs of beginners. Unlike the drop-in class, the participants will have registered, so you know who is coming. The series functions as a more in-depth way (rather than a single class) for people to see if the Alexander Technique could be useful for them in their life.

Adult continuing-education classes need to be designed with the knowledge that it is likely not everyone who signed up will make it to every class. Adults have a lot of competing priorities, thus absenteeism is usually not personal. One of my favorite examples of this—though it was about being late, rather than not coming at all—was of a woman with five children who was late to the class because she was walking by a shoe shop and realized she hadn't purchased a pair of shoes by herself in years. She bought some shoes, then came to class. I congratulated her on exercising her freedom of choice!

As noted in Part One, my perspective on the Alexander Technique derives from my own experience as an adult learner. While I took my first class in the Alexander Technique on the recommendation of a trusted mentor, once I was exposed to the work, I had a strong desire to learn it—because my acting got so much better. Consequently, in an introductory series, my aim is to create as many ways as I can for people to use the Alexander Technique to do the things they care about. Knowles's extensive research on what is effective for the adult learner consistently points to what he calls a "life-centered" orientation—a problem needs a solution or a skill needs development (Knowles *et al.*

2005, p.159). My introductory series design is designed to maximize the "life-centered" application of the Alexander Technique.

John Dewey, the American educational philosopher who studied with F.M. Alexander and wrote the introduction to F.M. Alexander's book *The Use of the Self*, is among the scholars Knowles discusses, particularly in relationship to learning from experience: "I assume that amid all uncertainties there is one permanent frame of reference: namely the organic connection between education and personal experience; or, that the new philosophy of education is committed to some kind of empirical and experimental philosophy" (Alexander 1984[1932], p.25).

The introductory series I teach most often is the one-week series for the University of Washington. It is slightly different than other adult continuing-education classes, in that this class is graded. (I grade based on participatory activities, not "coordination.") An extensive report on the class can be found in *Galvanizing Performance* (Madden and Juhl 2017, pp.220–260). After the first night of that class, I wrote:

> What was very exciting to note was the abundant and enthusiastic experimentation that was going on: Between 9:30 p.m. Monday and 5 p.m. on Tuesday, the Alexander Technique had been applied to an interview class, basketball, jogging and walking, piano, Suzuki training, driving, dancing, sit-ups and sitting, guitar, drumming, and monologues. Some of these represented their out-of-class experiments, but many more were moments in their life. (Madden and Juhl 2017, pp. 234–235)

That freedom to experiment is what I hope to foster in all my introductions.

Because introductory series can be of many durations, I offer some thoughts on sequencing that can be adapted to many structures.

The Emerged Order of Presentation

After teaching such introductions for many years, I have noticed that topics and needs seem to consistently arise in a particular order:

✓ Why study the Alexander Technique? What is the Alexander Technique?

- ✓ Our design—an introduction to how we work, including a first look at how thought manifests in our movement; bones; muscles; how the senses work; and more. The specific content is chosen based on the group and its needs.

- ✓ First experiments—introducing the AT Progression.

- ✓ Turns in applying the Alexander Technique.

As the practical application and experimentation provides more experience, questions about specific topics tend to appear in the following order:

- ✓ Concentration: What is whole-self thinking? Minking and thoving. Frank Pierce Jones's "integrated field of attention."

- ✓ Congruency: What is the appropriate amount of effort for the task? Coordination's role in supporting an excited state (as in performance) or a more subdued state (as in meditation).

- ✓ Omnisensory information: The role of sensory feedback, and how the senses work.

- ✓ Our biopsychosocial history: How the events and conditions of our lives create the patterns we have.

- ✓ Constructive planning—developing the AT Progression: Teaching the students how to use the AT Progression in their lives.

- ✓ Freedom of choice: Toward the end of the introductory series, there is often an aha! moment as people realize the implications of learning the Alexander Technique.

- ✓ Integration (F.M. Alexander's story) is the last class of the sequence.

I generally make sure that an introductory class has some version of F.M. Alexander's "Evolution of a Technique" chapter from *The Use of the Self.* If people have that story, in essence they have everything they need to continue studying. Most often, I give them a version I have created; the preponderance of good/bad/right/wrong in the original chapter puts people off.

Structuring the Series

If I am designing a ten-week series, each of these topics would have a featured night. The beginning of the class might present something about the special topic, either in a story or an activity of some sort. The bulk of each class, the middle section, is always experiment/studied rehearsed plan-oriented. As is generally true, all of these topics are part of every class; they receive special focus on their designated night.

Adapting this sequence to a five-class series involves combining foci. Following is how this might look.

Day One

✓ Why study the Alexander Technique? What is the Alexander Technique?

✓ First experiments

With a flavor of minking and thoving.

Day Two

✓ Our design

✓ Continuing experiments

With a flavor of omnisensory information.

Day Three

✓ Teaching the AT Progression

✓ Continuing experiments

With a flavor of analysis of activity.

Day Four

✓ Constructive planning and freedom of choice

✓ Continuing experiments

With a flavor of biopsychosocial.

Day Five

✓ Integration

With a flavor of simply means that I include a story, piece of information, or game that highlights the Alexander Technique's relationship to the idea.

Daily Structure Template

As in the introductory class and the drop-in class, an underlying design organizes the planning. The beginning invites the learning community to work together in a way that draws out desires and supports any theme of the day. The middle builds on this foundation, deliberately using the AT Progression in many experiments to develop studied rehearsed plans for life. The end validates, celebrates the work, encourages integration, and may have some return to the theme of the day. Table 25.1 is a simple template for planning.

Table 25.1 Class Planning Template

	Action Plan	Notes	Back-Up Plan
Preparation			
Beginning			
Middle			
End			
Evaluation			

Using this template, here is how I might plan a potential third class in a ten-class series (Table 25.2).

Third Night Class Planning–Teaching the AT Progression

Table 25.2 Sample Plan: Third Night

	Action Plan	Notes	Back-Up Plan
Preparation	Collect anatomy resources. Make AT Progression signs. Make AT Progression handouts.	I now have a permanent set of these signs and handouts.	If I am away from my materials, I will use parts of the teaching space to represent steps in the AT Progression.
Beginning	As everyone arrives, start teaching the components of the game that follows, without referencing the game. For example, using the Alexander Technique to walk, using the Alexander Technique to clap, using the Alexander Technique to nod. I will start this before the official start time. Teach a game in which sequence is important: "Walk, Clap, Nod." Ask students if they are bringing any questions or requests with them.	I usually start before the official start time because I prefer to have the room "in movement" as soon as possible. Marj often started early. In groups new to each other, it also facilitates the social interaction. See "Games Digest" for description and more options. I have many ways to ask the question "What do you want?"	As everyone arrives, begin quick turns in walking as you find out what questions they are bringing with them. Say the steps of the AT Progression as often as you can during this sequence.

	Action Plan	Notes	Back-Up Plan
Middle	Teach a few lessons as usual, verbally highlighting the steps in the process. Without teaching a lesson, talk about the progression, preferably writing on a board or an easel as you talk. Teach another lesson, and ask everyone to watch for the steps. Afterward, ask for responses. Introduce the Learning Structure game described in Chapter 5. I'll choose the more sedate version. I use the signs. A group of people is given a sign and their task is to watch the lesson from the perspective of that step in the process. After the lesson, the groups talk: Did they see that step? When? How many times did it repeat? Repeat the game through the rest of the sequence of the lessons, asking people to switch signs with each lesson.	Before doing a didactic piece, I am creating the context for why it is important. Writing, talking, and moving while you explain models many styles of learning. Interactive learning. Interaction and movement help learning. It also develops omniservation skills.	This can be an opportunity to tell F.M. Alexander's story via the AT Progression. Use one of the other versions of the Learning Structure game: the more aerobic or handout versions. I usually use the handout version of the Learning Structure game in the class that follows this one—as a review.
End	Give everyone a handout of the AT Progression, suggesting that they play with it between classes. If time permits, reprise the game we did at the beginning.	This can be quite fun to do because generally the skill level has increased.	Offer that Chapters 4 and 9 of my book *Integrative Alexander Technique Practice for Performing Artists: Onstage Synergy* (Madden 2014) cover this topic. I could also note F.M. Alexander's "Evolution of a Technique."
Evaluation	What did I actually do? What questions remain? What ideas does this give me for next time?		

The Daily Structure template is the backbone of the rest of the discussion around class and workshop planning. I include a column for back-up ideas because I have found it a good idea to have several back-ups. It is always important to note that just because you plan something, it may not be what you actually do. Having a well thought-out plan, however, is the necessary structure that helps us improvise within the teaching moment as needed.

Chapter 26

SHORT INTENSIVES

"Short intensives' are all-day workshops, weekend workshops, and multi-day (three to five days) workshops. These are concentrated opportunities for learning. I teach some workshops of this type at my Seattle studio, and this is the form in which I teach at most places where I am a guest teacher.

The essential planning structure is similar to that of the introductory series. Utilize the Daily Structure template for as many segments as there are sessions. For example, a weekend workshop typically is made up of four to five sessions, that is, Friday night, Saturday morning, Saturday afternoon, Sunday morning, Sunday afternoon = five plans. A daylong workshop with morning and afternoon sessions would be two plans. The plans for the individual sections are created in relationship to the overall goals of the event.

Returning to the AT Progression as the consistent guide in my work: Wanting, Recognizing, and Deciding happen in advance—as I either planned the intensive or agreed to teach the intensive. Prior to the event, I gather as much information as I can about what people want from the weekend. If I am organizing it, I do this at registration. If someone else is organizing the event, they may have a theme, which is inherently primary information. If the event is without a theme, I often ask my hosts to solicit desires from the registrants if possible. I explain that having this information ahead of time helps me honor everyone's time by planning appropriately. Not everyone will answer, but any information I receive helps.

Although having them ahead of time is more efficient, I can collect the wants when people arrive.

Sessions in Short Intensive

I offer a fictional example first. The second and third examples are actual teaching plans from previous workshops. If you compare what the students asked for with what I chose to do, you get a glimpse of my planning process. These descriptions do not detail what took place within the particular individual lessons (turns). While I can extrapolate what questions were arising from those turns, I generally don't take notes on the turns themselves. Note that many of the games mentioned can be found in "Games Digest."

Example One

The first offering is a fictitious account of the first session of a weekend workshop in my studio, allowing me to make the descriptions and choices more transparent. Although I draw upon history of real people and the requests they might make in this setting, the workshop depicted has never taken place.

Before the workshop, I gather information about what people would like to explore. This group's composite response includes monologues, reading aloud, a dance step, a difficult communication task, and working at a computer.

Session One
Beginning
All of these participants have met before and so are really part of an ongoing learning cohort. It is evening and all will have had a full day, so I select a simple game to start: a Slinky-like spring toy that rolls along your arm and can be passed from arm to arm, person to person around the circle. It is fun, the motion is a bit beautiful, and the activity gives the group a few minutes to play together. While the requests for the workshop on their face seem quite different, all are related to communication. This game wakes up playful communication. My back-up idea, since they already know the Alexander Technique, is a round of walks.

Middle
Playing with mirror exercises to continue warming up the Alexander Technique and communication with sound and movement experiments,

including breathing as well as the arm and leg motion that we need for dancing, speaking, and the computer.

Activities and turns emphasizing using the Alexander Technique to invite communication, noting what is possible, constructive, within your control, and ecological. In collecting requests, I have noted that perhaps some of the interference people are describing might be coming from communication plans that don't meet the change plan criteria.

Back-up ideas include a review of breathing, potentially by teaching a sound warm-up; a review of how limb movement relates to the central coordination—including anatomy and movement (particularly for the dance and the computer).

End

Returning to the spring toy from the beginning. On the first round, saying something you've learned from the night—either from your own turn or someone else's; on the second round, voicing your wish for the next morning's class.

Example Two

This is a real-life report of a continuing education intensive for Alexander Technique teachers.

Session One

Beginning

In this case, the wants were not expressed ahead of time. To begin the event, I offered my then-nascent quest—using an invented word as the verb to represent the action of leaving behind our old plan and inviting our natural coordination to return, so we can do what we are doing. We picked a verb—*rakusa*. My plan was to follow this up with using the Alexander Technique to walk outside because we were in nature and I always love to make the connection between Alexander Technique and nature. (It was raining so we did this inside.) Following that, I collected their wants: group work, communication, fear of leadership, singing, how to introduce Alexander Technique to a group of musicians, integrated Alexander Technique practice, more about groups, dance, games in teaching, using the technique for daily life activities. This led us into a break.

Middle

During the break, I considered the wants and how to start addressing them. I decided on a daily activity round (and noted a back-up idea—a part-of-the-body moving round). By *round*, I mean that everyone has a short turn doing something. Our evening time is limited, and simply going around the circle (as long as everyone knows they can pass) is faster than asking for turn volunteers. I announce it as a short round to orient people's expectations toward a glimpse of a new idea rather than an in-depth exploration. I consider this sort of "round" a game. This is particularly useful in the first session of an extended workshop. Everyone begins their process, the learning community starts to coalesce, and it is low key. For the people interested in group teaching, a "round of turns" offers an example of a group process; the people looking to integrate Alexander Technique with life, music, dance, and communication were encouraged to select relevant activities; and I was modeling leadership.

End

As we were in a town that had a fairy tale associated with it, I made up a game to go with the story.

Session Two

Beginning

The next morning, I taught the group as I would a beginning Alexander Technique class to answer in action their questions about teaching and group teaching. I chose the act of reaching to a real or imagined musical instrument as the demonstration activity to address some questions about the use of hands in teaching and how to teach an introductory class to musicians. In my notes, I chose particular things to emphasize, based on the questions from the night before. Before a coffee break, I asked for questions.

Middle

My notes say, "If you didn't have a turn yesterday, here is an opportunity," indicating that I didn't make it through the daily activity round the night before. This can happen. The overall plan is individual turns, beginning with those who haven't yet had one. As a back-up, I list potential games, all of which are those that build omniservation skills, a necessity for group teaching.

End

I have several pages of questions that I solicited or came up at the close. In between each session, I note items I've looked up or want to follow up on in the following session.

Session Three

Note that this report skips two sessions ahead. The planning page for this session illustrates that I take time management seriously. Many of the plans recorded in my notebooks include a timeline. Omniservation skills (I called them "observation skills" at the time) were a prominent question in this group.

Beginning

9 a.m.: Starting with walks (noting that a new participant arrived that morning who was completely new to the Alexander Technique, so I was also using these walks to introduce the work to her). Once everyone arrived, we played with one walk using the Alexander Technique, one walk with a slump, one walk with the Alexander Technique, one with a slump, then played back and forth while also noticing what was happening with everyone else.

9:15: Review the schedule for the day, which alternated turns with group activities to train omniservation skills.

Middle

9:25: "Circle Omniservation" game

9:40: Activities/turns 1, 2, 3, 4

10:10: Mirrors, another omniservation game

10:20: Activities/turns 5, 6

10:30: Break

10:45: Reaching for something, watching your hand as you do it (another teaching skill)

11:00: "Elephant," also an omniservation game

11:05: Activities 7, 8, 9, 10

11:30: "Change Three Things" omniservation game

11:35: Rest of turns/activities

End

11:50: Ending game, if have time (I bet there wasn't—it's always better to have more planned than you need.)

Example Three

A mixed group of people learning the Alexander Technique for personal use, with some interested in teaching.

Session One
Beginning
A series of activities, leading to meeting each other:

- ✓ Using the Alexander Technique, reach for the paper.

- ✓ Using the Alexander Technique, reach for the pencil.

- ✓ Using the Alexander Technique, watch your hands and fingers as you move the pencil.

- ✓ Using the Alexander Technique, turn your head to look at someone.

- ✓ Using the Alexander Technique, draw a picture of that person, while continuing to look at them (not at the paper).

I solicited their wants, which included: arms, teaching, mental and emotional comfort, more arms, relationships, archery, tension, how to teach without right/wrong judgment, reciting a poem, coordinating while afraid, and drawing.

Middle
A series of initial activities and turns.

End
I didn't note the end, although one of the back-up ideas listed was a game I had learned from people teaching horseback riding—"Horses

and Riders." Because game elements can address arms, teaching, and communication, it would have been a good choice.

Session Two
Beginning
I talked about the Alexander Technique's insistence on freedom of choice, then told a story about something that had happened to me on the way to the workshop relevant to freedom of choice (also addressing mental/emotional comfort, tension, nonjudgment, and fear). Storytelling can be an inviting start to a workshop session.

Middle

- ✓ "Chair Freedom of Choice" game

- ✓ Activities/turns

- ✓ "Chair Maze" game

- ✓ Activities/turns

End
I invented a game that combined using the arms, choice, and coordinating to the unknown. The latter clearly emerged from questions regarding mental/emotional comfort and tension. My notes seem to indicate that the unknown was associated, in particular, with fear. Here is the game.

"TREASURE HUNT WITH PAPERS"
On a sheet of paper, I had everyone write names of places to go on vacation. Next, they exchanged the papers with someone else, considering the "how" of the movement itself and inviting the other person along while offering them the paper, doing the same to receive the paper. Then, I had everyone close their eyes as I hid the papers all over the room.

When they opened their eyes, I asked them to use the Alexander Technique to look for the papers and to pick them up as they found them, then to use the Alexander Technique to see where they got to go on vacation. My intention was to create something to do that would involve something pleasant happening in the unknown—their surprise vacation spot. The game enfolded elements associated with all of Friday night's wants as well.

> *I don't think I've played this game anywhere else, as it was specific to that group. Now that I've rediscovered it in my notebook, it might appear again.*

My hope is that, throughout these reports, you can recognize me saying "yes" to all the participants' wants, calling on all of my information and experience and letting everything dance together to create a workshop. In doing this, I am able to address questions both indirectly and directly. What I find is that this meticulously planned, yet organic process, inspires questions to arise that are just "below the surface" of the activities or questions that are asked.

Chapter 27

LONGER-RANGE COURSES

Take the Daily Structure template and multiply it by the number of sessions you have. Then consider what the intent of the workshop is—from your perspective and from the student perspective. What steps do you imagine will create that overall journey? How does the number of steps within this arc match the number of sessions you have?

In longer-range courses—residentials, university terms, teacher training programs—we need to plan from both the perspective of the end result and that of the current needs considered in relationship to the desired end result.

Designing from the Desired End Result

As an example, what if you are teaching an Alexander Technique course for public speakers with the desired end result that in the last of the ten sessions, everyone gives a three-minute speech using the Alexander Technique? What steps do you need to accomplish that?

Starting the planning from the desired end could look like this:

✓ Session 10: Individual speeches

✓ Session 9: Using the Alexander Technique for different types of rehearsals

✓ Session 8: Continuing Session 7 topics, adding exploration of memorization

✓ Session 7: Using the Alexander Technique to analyze performance circumstances and to rehearse; particular attention on how to use the Alexander Technique to respond to perceived obstacles

✓ Session 6: Opening-sentence rehearsals

✓ Session 5: Using the Alexander Technique to choose material that you have a desire to communicate

✓ Session 4: The Alexander Technique and inviting the audience to be with you while you are with them

✓ Session 3: The Alexander Technique and breath and speech in more depth

✓ Session 2: The Alexander Technique and our design, applied to walking, talking, or a simple activity of their choice

✓ Session 1: Introducing the Alexander Technique, with individual introductions to the group as the sample activity (including inviting us to be with you while you are with us and intending to include invitation in every class)

In creating this imaginary class design, I filled in Sessions 10 to 6 first, then went back to Session 1 and worked back up to Session 5. You need to know where you are going in order to plan the sequence.

The next step would be to start filling in the daily plans. In this case, because I imagine this as a class that is also introducing the Alexander Technique, I would match the outline above with the sequence of learning Alexander Technique I had devised for the introductory series:

✓ Session 1: Why study the Alexander Technique? What is the Alexander Technique?

✓ Session 2: Introduction to our design

✓ Session 3: First experiments; introducing the AT Progression

✓ Session 4: Concentration (minking and thoving)

✓ Session 5: Congruency (including beginning analysis of activity)

✓ Session 6: Omnisensory information

✓ Session 7: Biopsychosocial

✓ Session 8: Constructive planning—developing the AT Progression

✓ Session 9: Freedom of choice

✓ Session 10: Integration (F.M. Alexander's story), the last class of the sequence

Comparing the first set of topics with the second set looks like a complementary match. To plan each class, you would consider both formulations. Note that, at this point, only the first daily planning class can be completely planned. I could map out potential beginnings and endings for each of the days based on the topics. However, because I don't yet know the people and their particular wants and desires, it is impossible to plan the middle beyond intending to do a variety of activities and turns, many related to speaking. To fully plan each session, I need the interaction with the students—they are co-creators of the class.

A shorthand chart of the elements that generate complete planning is provided in Table 27.1.

Table 27.1 Longer-Range Class Planning

Session	Class Topic	Alexander Technique Topic	Student Input
1	Alexander Technique and speech*	Why/what is the Alexander Technique?	What brings them to class?
2	Alexander Technique and our design*	Our design	What took place in the last class; student responses/questions since last class
3	Alexander Technique and breath/speech in more depth*	AT Progression, experiments	As above
4	Inviting the audience to be with you	Concentration	As above
5	Choosing material*	Congruency	As above
6	Opening sentence rehearsals*	Omnisensory information	As above
7	Performance circumstances*	Biopsychosocial	As above

cont.

Session	Class Topic	Alexander Technique Topic	Student Input
8	Continuing performance and adding memorization*	Constructive planning	As above
9	Using the Alexander Technique for different kinds of rehearsals*	Freedom of choice	As above
10	Individual speeches*	Integration	As above

*The asterisk is intended to remind me that I want to include something about inviting the audience to be with you while you are with them every week. If we use the Alexander Technique to include this from the beginning, then people are ready to welcome the audience (this is a preventive for what some call "stage fright").

From the chart for this fictitious class, an idea emerges: Have the class create a ten-step activity, then do one step together each week. I would be inclined to make this a moving activity in contrast to speaking, one that is playful and perhaps frivolous in contrast to their serious goal of speaking. In session one, we'll have everyone create a group human sculpture together, somewhat literally becoming a learning cohort. We'll use the Alexander Technique to facilitate efficiency in any of the shapes they come up with, then do it again, inviting everyone to be with us while making it (practicing a communication skill via movement). Each subsequent week, we'll make a new sculpture, then recreate the previous weeks' sculptures. We'll use the Alexander Technique to move back and forth among them in a dance of sorts, inviting people to be with us while we are with them. We are exercising integrative Alexander Technique skills in communication and movement. Through play, we are evolving a parallel development process to the sequential public speaking process, indirectly reinforcing the learning with a visible weekly result.

Having the big picture—the end—creates the ability to consider the means.

Multi-Year Courses

In multi-year courses, the planning comprises both institutional and highly individual goals. There is an arc of intention, which may be generally defined by an individual with the intent of continuous learning or specifically defined by the needs of a profession—such as in an arts training program or when someone decides to learn to teach the Alexander Technique. The arc of planning ranges longer and is constantly renegotiated per the actual experience of the individual or those in the course. Although the variables are many, the questions in planning are still the same: Where are we intending to go? Which ways seem to lead us there? And what alternate ways might lead us there?

I teach multi-year courses for individuals, in the three-year Professional Actor Training Program at the University of Washington, and in an apprentice-style teacher training at my studio in Seattle. Key in each of these situations is a constant monitoring—from informal to formal—of the arc of intention and the ongoing emergent means-whereby.

Chapter 28

THE PLETHORA OF TEACHING EVENTS

As Alexander Technique teachers, our range of teaching possibilities is rich. I have taught in barns, corporate offices, art studios; I have occasionally been backstage during a performance; I have taught exceedingly large groups and many different kinds of groups. Many of my colleagues have taught in situations I haven't yet explored; the possibilities are limited perhaps only by time. All the skills and processes we have covered thus far can mix, match, and combine to respond to many circumstances. This chapter considers a few of them.

The Private Lesson

I could accurately call this section "The Smallest Group." For me, teaching one person is essentially the same as teaching all kinds of groups. In a sense, it is similar to the drop-in class or the multi-year course, in that, although you know who is coming, you don't know exactly what request your student will have. It may look like a specialty class if your student is examining a particular goal; recently, for example, I was helping someone prepare for a TED talk. The planning I do for private lessons happens in the moment as I hear what questions a student is bringing to our learning playground that day. Because I have done a lot of formal planning, my facility for improvisational planning continues to grow.

A Few Additional Thoughts

Even though there is only one student in the lesson, you often need to switch activities just as if there were more people in the class. This most frequently happens when the student asks a question, and through their explorations using the Alexander Technique, successfully resolves it, essentially completing a turn. This may happen within the first few minutes of a half-hour lesson. Rather than repeating the successful turn immediately, you might want some integration time. Your choices are similar to what you might do in a group: change to another activity, or play a game, or ask what else they would like to explore, or perhaps follow up on something from a previous lesson.

The private lesson offers an opportunity for in-depth exploration of a particular project. Many performers who study with me in group settings also want private lessons so that they can develop a dance, monologue, or concerto. These lessons, in essence, become Alexander Technique-infused rehearsals.

When an individual has come to you for private lessons over time, the strength of the relationship along with the many experiments often results in a lot of shorthand communication. Both of you are aware of the arc of learning you have been traveling together. At the same time, we as humans are always changing. The person arriving is a lot like the person you saw last time—and is also new. As are you.

Online Teaching

The first lessons I taught in which I was not in the room with the student were by telephone. A man in Texas, having no teacher nearby, asked for phone conferences with me over several weeks. I was initially dubious, as the only information I could glean was how he described his experience and how his voice sounded from the ideas I offered. Nonetheless, he reported learning.

While many of my colleagues are teaching online more than I, I am happy to teach in this medium. When I first taught in the online environment, I already knew that it was absolutely possible to talk someone through a lesson, using omniservation and the ability to verbalize what I see. The more precise, the better. My ability to demonstrate is also a necessary asset, certainly possible via the device's camera.

I continue to note that many people today learn best by seeing what I do. The amount of time we spend interacting with the virtual world through the internet has trained people how to learn this way. What is of paramount importance to be effective in the online teaching environment is the ability to, while seeing small, two-dimensional people on the screen, imagine students life-sized and three-dimensional. In addition, I regularly ask my online students to change angles in relationship to their device as needed in order to get a more complete look. In this environment, using words that emphasize dimensionality is skillful.

Initially, the people I was teaching online were people I had taught "live." The first time I taught someone I had never met in same time-same space, I was curious to see if it would eliminate a question I usually get in early lessons. Sure enough, several months into our sessions, he made a beautiful change in what he was doing at his desk. He exclaimed into the monitor, "Yes, but how do I do that myself?" I pointed out that as he was across oceans and thousands of miles away, I was pretty sure he did it himself! Then, we reviewed the steps he had just gone through so that he knew he could replicate the process that created the change.

I have taught a young child in an online learning environment for several years (occasionally supplemented by in-person lessons), and it works beautifully. The medium makes this work available to more people than ever before, and teachers and students alike will all continue to learn how to use it better and better.

Very Large Groups

Like the special-interest workshops that follow, very large groups generally have a particular purpose—they are for a particular organization, school, or event. Clarifying what the stakeholders want from the introduction guides the choice of material. If they are simply looking for an introduction to the Alexander Technique, then the first part of my introduction where I teach people the AT Progression prior to using any tactile communication works well. Following that, demonstration lessons with as many people as time permits is an option. It is also possible to lead the whole group through a pertinent activity step by step.

As always, it's meaningful to select an activity that matches what the group does in some way. I also like finding a small prop or toy that somehow relates to who these students are. For instance, I was teaching a group of people associated with the paper industry, so I brought small blow-up balls made out of paper. I knew some of the group wanted to get information about speaking, so blowing up the balls as the introductory activity started integrating the Alexander Technique with breathing. I wondered if having something made of paper would add another resonance—it seemed to, as many of them really examined the paper itself. For another group, whose central theme involved celebrity, I brought a bunch of second-hand bowties. People remember small touches—it adds a playful sensory element.

People can learn the process of the Alexander Technique and use it themselves without a direct lesson, without tactile communication. Your ability to model and to invite people to be with you as you model the process of change is always important; in very large groups, it is your major ally in teaching. Your belief and trust that everyone in the room is capable of making the choices you are offering is paramount. Watching a room of 100 people the first time they hear about the head–spine relationship—and discovering they can choose the quality of that relationship—is a wonder to behold.

Special-Interest Workshops

What I am calling "special-interest workshops" are those organized for you by other individuals or a group with a specific topic that they are interested in. For example, a singing teacher may have me come and do an introduction for their studio.

A few things to consider regarding special-interest workshops:

- A clear preparation that clarifies your role is vital—you are the Alexander Technique expert, they are the experts in what they do.

- The selection of introductory material relative to why one might study the Alexander Technique, ideally is tailored specifically for the group.

- The selection of activities to use in introducing the Alexander Technique, ideally relates to their interest.

- Research—you are more effective if you have done some research about what they care about.

I define my boundaries: I have yet to make a sound on a regular flute; my computer programming skills have yet to exist; I have what they call a "deep seat" when on a horse but am unpracticed at actually riding. When asked to teach any of these groups, what I have said before—your student always knows more about what is happening in a lesson than you do—is demonstrably true. My job isn't to know their specialty, but rather to help them coordinate to their expertise and desires.

Research! I am teaching a talented young ice skater and have been watching the ISU Grand Prix finals to gather information. Amid writing this chapter, I remembered that I was helping someone use Alexander Technique to do the Bird Dog Core Exercise and a question arose, so I paused my writing to look it up. For corporate workshops, the organizers work with me to ensure that I have the information I need to make the most effective presentation for these particular employees.

Occasionally, I might take a class in the area of expertise. A group was interested in creating an Alexander Technique course for belly dancers and asked me to help design it. I had little idea what belly dancers needed or experienced, but I knew a prominent belly dance teacher lived in Seattle. Looking her up, I was delighted to discover that she had an introductory evening coming up. I was the only one who signed up for the class. She chose to teach it anyway: my workshop turned into a very long private lesson. She even ran overtime, bringing out all sorts of scarves and bells and belts—I almost had to beg to leave. Her teaching skills were great; I enjoyed experiencing her expertise and got tons of information for designing my workshop.

Teaching the Alexander Technique alongside great teachers of other disciplines is another way I have built my resources for specialty workshops. I have been lucky to teach the Alexander Technique with dressage teachers, many singing and voice teachers, several world-class choreographers, some fabulous Suzuki (theatre) teachers, and acting and stage combat teachers. Plus many more.

Another source for key information are students who are experts in their fields. I have been known to say in a lesson, "You can thank the pianists I have taught before you for that piece of information." Or, "I learned to describe it that way from a painter I taught." If I am teaching in a group of experts, I regularly call on them to comment on each other's lessons. Their feedback to their colleague is more precise in relationship to the field, and, incidentally, I learn more about what is important to them. For instance, I regularly call on other musicians to offer feedback when a musician makes a change, particularly if their concern is intonation or timbre. While my specificity in reporting musical change has gotten much better from teaching musicians, I know that the assessment from another musician offers detail beyond my own and may be more credible.

Knowing as much as you can about the specialty helps you tailor your messages so they are most on point, as well as to select as your demonstration activity something that is immediately useful to the group (Table 28.1).

Table 28.1 Special-Interest Activities

If your group are...	The activity could be...
dancers	pliés
instrumentalists	opening their case
singers	humming
computer programmers	solving a coding puzzle
artists	drawing
psychology students	reading and taking notes
sales personnel	shaking hands
martial artists	the first movement of their form
hikers	going up steps (or a hill if one is nearby)

And so forth…

One of the greatest things you can do for your student is to immediately integrate the Alexander Technique with the things they love and care about. And one of my great joys in teaching Alexander Technique is the opportunity to visit worlds I would otherwise never have a glimpse of. The range of what humans enjoy and value seems endless.

Chapter 29

GAMES DIGEST

Spotlighting games as a teaching tool comes naturally to me. Games have the potential to illuminate how to use the Alexander Technique in real-life situations. Students play freely with choices they might want to consider in life, testing them before accepting them in their daily routine. Games operate outside the spheres of necessity and right/wrong, facilitating experimentation. Bob Fagen, an expert in animal play behavior, suggested that humans share many of the reasons bears play: "In a world continuously presenting unique challenges and ambiguity, play prepares these bears for an evolving planet" (Brown 2009, p.29).

While I think every Alexander Technique class and lesson is play, games are even more obviously play. My theatre training contributes to my deep appreciation of the value of games in learning, also providing a deep well of game resources.

Games...

- Help create a learning community.
- Introduce a playful approach to learning.
- Illustrate/embody concepts.
- Include every member of a group.
- Change the mood or tempo.
- Mimic situations people find stressful so they can practice new responses.

- Indirectly offer a new idea when someone is on a learning "edge of comfort."

- Explore anatomy and movement in action.

- Rehearse new studied rehearsed plans.

- Uncover questions that someone didn't know to ask.

I offer a collection of games in the following section. Some of these games are adapted from various sources, some are games I learned in my theatre classes, and some are games I made up along the way. Sources for games are abundant; your own childhood games are a great starting point. At one Alexander Technique International Annual Conference, the International Committee sponsored a workshop in which we taught childhood games from each of our different cultures. These games gave us a fascinating glimpse into each other's values, while offering a wealth of potential teaching tools.

Some Curiosities about Games

People often learn something different than you thought the game would teach. I go with what they learn. And then find another way to teach what I intended to teach. You need to be attentive to how people are responding. In one workshop in Germany, a participant was clearly in distress as we played the group juggling game. The game had reminded him of some unpleasant childhood experiences with balls. We used it as an opportunity to rehearse responding to balls with coordination, yet he remained unsettled. At lunchtime, I walked past a store that had juggling supplies, and saw foam animals. In moments, I was in the store buying a pig, cow, and sheep. When we returned from lunch, I brought out my purchases and asked the participant if he'd like to play group juggling with the foam animals. He was delighted—I can almost still hear his glee at throwing cows around!

Creating Your Own Games

More often than serving up a set game, I find myself making up a game that matches the needs of the particular moment. Some of the following games began as games I needed for a specific group and have now become part of my "stock of choices." Creating a game is akin to storytelling, in that it begins with a problem; has a beginning, middle, and end; and its process reveals something pertinent to the learning.

A game I use now that began as something I made up in the moment is the "Create a Spine" game. I was teaching an introductory series, and some people missed the class that offered some basic anatomy. I needed to catch them up, yet wanted to offer something that wasn't a rerun for the participants who were at the first session. Likely I also thought we needed something active for a change of pace.

My ability to make up games comes in part from consistently experiencing the structure of existing games in acting and Alexander Technique classes. As I used these preset structures, I learned how to create my own. If you make up a game, and it doesn't work, that is okay—it is just a game. This also gives you a real moment to model that mistakes are perfectly welcome.

Following are some of the many games I use in teaching. My intent is to offer a representative sample to get you started. They are listed alphabetically.

12 DOT NAMETAGS

Participants: Any number

Supplies: Pens, markers, or crayons. Small cards dotted with 12 roughly evenly spaced dots as follows:

•	•	•	•
•	•	•	•
•	•	•	•

Source: Cathy Madden (I was in a teaching studio in Zurich with many paintings on the wall, all based on the same pattern of dots filled in many different ways, which inspired this game)

Description

Making these nametags is a possibility for the first class. Everyone receives a card with dots as they arrive, and pens or markers are made available.

Give any three instructions about how to color the 12 dots, such as:

1. Use two colors.

2. Make one line.

3. Draw a triangle.

Then draw your name on the resultant drawing.

While everyone follows the same instructions, all the cards end up looking different. As everyone finishes, I invite them to share their nametags with each other, pointing out that they are all different and all "right."

How I Use This Game

Particularly if I use this game to start a first class, it signals that the learning environment is playful and interactive. Because every card turns out different and every card is right, the activity exemplifies that I think in the "yes" (rather than in terms of right or wrong).

The nametags are a gradual way for people to meet each other: what begins as an individual task becomes shared, providing a gradual sequence toward group participation.

A WHAT? A WHAT?

Participants: At least 7

Supplies: Two small props—for example, two different-colored Koosh balls would work well

Source: Adapted from *More New Games* (Fluegelman 1981, p.73)

Description

Everyone sits in a circle. One person starts the game by passing an object to the person to their right, naming it imaginatively. The general script for this game is this:

Leader: "This is a(n) _____."

Person to their right (hereafter Person A): "A what?"

Leader: "A(n) _____."

Person A: "Oh, a(n) _____."

The rhythm of the script is important.

For example, if the Leader named the object a kumquat, the sequence would go:

Leader: "This is a kumquat." (*indicating the object*)

Person A: (to Leader) "A what?"

Leader: "A kumquat."

Person A: "Oh, a kumquat." (*taking the object*)

The sequence continues around the circle as follows:

Person A (to the person to their right, hereafter Person B): "This is a kumquat." (*indicating the object*)

Person B (*to Person A*): "A what?"

Person A (*to Leader*): "A what?"

Leader (*to Person A*): "A kumquat."

Person A (*to Person B*): "A kumquat."

Person B: "Oh, a kumquat." (*taking the object*)

Person B then tells the person to their right (who becomes Person C), "This is a kumquat," and play continues as before, the object gradually making its way around the circle.

Once you rehearse the pattern once around the circle, you can play the game, adding the second object. To begin the game, the Leader names and starts both objects around—one to the right, one to the left—in immediate succession using the same script (while giving each object a different name). You now have two objects with different names traveling around the circle in opposite directions, using the same general script. As you can imagine, complication and excitement occurs as the objects pass each other.

How I Use This Game

The key to the game is to do each task one at a time while using the Alexander Technique, creating an operational practice of whole-self thinking. Because it has steps, it is a way to emphasize the step-by-step process of the means-whereby we do things. As with all of the games that involve some kind of complication, it can be useful for groups who want to use the Alexander Technique to cope with intricate or thorny situations.

AURA OR PERIPERSONAL SPACE VARIATIONS

Participants: 2 or more, done in pairs

Source: Adapted from *The New Games Book* (Fluegelman 1976, p.37); I learned similar games in acting classes

Description

Two people stand opposite one another and hold their hands out toward each other, intentionally reaching into each other's peripersonal space. One person closes their eyes and turns themselves in a circle about three times. Then, with eyes still closed, they seek to return to their original orientation to their partner.

Eyes Open Variation

Two people stand opposite one another with the intention simply to be with each other, again consciously choosing to be in each other's peripersonal space. Then they gradually start to move away from each other, intending to stay connected, moving toward and away from each other as needed to keep the connection going.

Large Group Variation

Send one person out of the room. The remaining people, as silently as possible, move as a group to a section of the room. The person is assisted back to the room with eyes closed, and has the job of finding the rest of the group. The group, for their part, silently invites the person to walk in their direction.

How I Use This Game

I generally include this game in a performers workshop to explicate the idea of invitation in performance. It also appears in group teaching workshops to develop the skill of inviting a group to be with you while you are with them. It sometimes helps to explain that we have a spatial sense.

Note that I don't ever actually call this game "Aura," although that is what the source text calls it.

CHAIR FREEDOM OF CHOICE

Participants: 1 to 500

Supplies: A chair for each person

Source: Cathy Madden

Description

Arrange the chairs in a circle. Each person stands behind their chair, with the goal of walking to the center. Before they move, everyone decides whether they will go to the center of the circle by going to the right or left of their chair. Everyone has the option to remain where they are.

We do several rounds of this. At the moment when they decide to walk to center, I coach them to use the Alexander Technique to choose again: Alexander Technique to the right, Alexander Technique to the left, or Alexander Technique to stay where they are. I encourage people to experiment with all the choices—sometimes doing what they intended, sometimes changing to the other side of the chair, sometimes choosing to stay behind their chair—using the Alexander Technique to carry through all the decisions.

Variation

If you have a garden that has pathways forking into right and left choices, it is lovely to play this out in nature.

How I Use This Game

This game gives a practical version of the process F.M. Alexander describes in *The Use of the Self*, in which he renews his freedom of choice, knowing he could speak, continue doing what he was doing, or do something else.

CHAIR MAZE

Participants: As few as 1; more fun with many

Supplies: Enough chairs to create a maze

Source: Cathy Madden

Description

Create a maze using chairs and/or other available furniture pieces. One side of the construction is designated the entrance, the other is the exit.

Variation One

Everyone in the group goes through the maze with the instruction to do so in a different way than everyone before them. The teaching point is that every passage is different, and all of them are "right."

Variation Two

Ask people to renew the Alexander Technique each time they change direction in the maze. It is important to me that they don't actually stop at these change points, but simply renew their wish for themselves as they continue to walk through the maze.

Variation Three

Ask a couple of people to be in the maze as "obstacles," trying to prevent people from getting through. The task is to use the Alexander Technique when confronted by an obstacle.

How I Use This Game

Each variation has a slightly different teaching point, as noted in the descriptions. Overall, the game is a great group exploration. If the group has been sitting for a while, it gets everyone up and moving to make the maze (creating opportunities for Alexander Technique lessons about lifting and moving objects). People get to watch each other solving the puzzles the maze presents in a variety of different ways. It is practice at using external cues to invite yourself to use the Alexander Technique; and because the cue is a change in direction, it is widely applicable to daily life.

CHANGE THREE THINGS

Participants: 2 or more, done in pairs

Source: Learned in an acting class

Description

Two people stand opposite each other omniserving each other. After a few minutes, Person A turns away from their partner and closes their eyes. Person B changes three things about themselves. When Person B is ready, Person A is invited to turn around, open their eyes, and try to spot the three differences.

How I Use This Game

This is an easy and fun omniservation game.

CIRCLE OMNISERVATION

Participants: Best with 7 or more

Source: From my theatre training

Description

The group makes a circle, and one person is sent outside the room. Someone in the circle volunteers to be the Leader and, staying in the circle, everyone plays "Follow the Leader," with the Leader subtly shifting from one movement/gesture to another. The person outside the room comes back in and stands in the center of the circle, omniserving the game in hopes of identifying who the Leader is— while the rest of the participants do their best to disguise the Leader. When the person in the middle guesses correctly, the Leader becomes the player who leaves the room, and you play again. Repeat as many times as you like.

How I Use This Game

This game is particularly helpful in omniserving sequence of movement. It also enables someone to play with being a leader in a nonthreatening way.

COUNTING TO 21

Participants: At least 2; more is better

Source: Many people attribute this game to Peter Brook, who says he didn't make it up

Description

The object is for the group to count to 21. The counting is done by one person at a time, but the order is not predetermined. If two people say the same number at the same time, the group starts over.

How I Use This Game

This is another game in which the learning community has a puzzle to solve that is likely to involve "mistakes," giving everyone an opportunity to experience mistake-making as a safe, even fun or funny, event. The game calls for what Frank Pierce Jones called an "integrated field of attention."

ELEPHANT

Participants: Best with 10 or more

Source: Various sources

Description

The group sits in a circle, with one person volunteering to be in the center. The person in the center (Person A) points to a person in the circle (Person B). Person B moves their arms with two fists together in front of their nose to create an elephant trunk. The two people on either side of Person B move their hand closest to Person B to Person B's ear, creating a larger elephant ear. At whatever speed they prefer, Person A points to different Person Bs, in turn. Each new Person B makes the elephant's trunk, and the people beside that person make the ears.

If someone misses their cue or makes the "wrong" elephant part, they become the person in the center.

How I Use This Game

This games builds omniservation skills because you need to respond rapidly to stimuli. It may be useful for people looking to use the Alexander Technique to learn a new response to speed and/or what they perceive as stress.

EVERYONE DO THIS!

Participants: As many as you have

Source: Cathy Madden

Description

This game arises when a person in the group asks a question about an activity common to our everyday lives—like washing your face. Then, everyone in the group gets up and experiments with how each of them might apply the Alexander Technique to face washing. It is fun to explore the variations everyone comes up with.

How I Use This Game

Because opportunities to create external cues to use the Alexander Technique serve everyone, anytime a daily activity comes up in class, I like to take the opportunity to amplify the cue.

This is also a precursor to the Round Robin (Variation 3) game.

FINGER PUPPET MONSTERS AND FLYING CHICKENS

Description

A longtime student, Patt Schwab, introduced me to a variety of teaching toys. The focus of her career as a speaker is humor in the workplace. She regularly traveled with rubber chickens in her carry-on baggage. One time, she was transporting rubber chickens that screeched when they decompressed. When called aside for special security at the airport, she suddenly realized that, when her carry-on was opened, there would be a loud screeching noise! She quickly explained—all went well.

I have a variety of finger puppet monsters and little versions of the flying chickens in my studio to use when I need them.

The finger puppet monsters are particularly good for helping someone tame any particularly pesky critical voices. The idea is to decide that the critical voice is coming from the finger puppet monster—correctly identifying the critical voice as external to self, and using a bit of humor to put it in perspective.

The rubber chickens are a humorous way to bring perspective to anger. Anger is a perfectly useful human emotion. We need it. Sometimes, we also need a way to express anger—and rubber chickens are an option. Patt encourages managers in corporations to have a rubber chicken handy for when someone gets frustrated: they can come into the manager's office, ask for the chicken, and bang it around for a while. I find having rubber chickens around is a useful reminder that anger can be perfect.

FOLLOWING THE BALL

Participants: At least 2; can be many more

Supplies: One large exercise ball or Swiss ball

Source: Cathy Madden

Description

Players sit in a circle (or opposite each other, if just two). They pass the ball around the group randomly. As players see the ball coming toward them, they use the Alexander Technique to move their fingers to the ball in such a way that their hand shapes to the ball, to follow the movement of the ball, and then to redirect it to someone else.

How I Use This Game

This game develops skills in using finger/hand/arm movement for Alexander Technique teaching and other purposes.

GROUP ART CREATION

Participants: Any number

Supplies: Portable objects, ideally from nature

Source: Cathy Madden

Description

I created this game arose from a desire to invite the creative process into the Alexander Technique studio in a way that was accessible to everyone—particularly those who considered themselves non-performers. Whenever possible, this activity takes place out of doors and is the first one of the day.

As you think about your desires for the day, you find something (a rock, stick, flower, pencil…) that represents your desire and take it to a selected spot in the teaching area. Everyone contributes their objects, placing them in any relationship to the others to make a group piece of art. If you are doing a multi-day workshop, you could add to your artwork every day. We do this each year at my Friday Harbor residential workshop. It was fun to return for the 2017 residential and be greeted by remnants of the 2016 sculptural project!

How I Use This Game

This game invites creative thinking while awakening desire for the day of learning.

GROUP JUGGLING

Participants: At least 4

Supplies: At least three juggling balls or other small objects of some kind, ideally like Koosh balls that won't bounce far away

Source: Adapted from *More New Games* (Fluegelman 1981, p.61)

Description

Make a circle and select someone to throw the ball first. The group first creates a pattern by throwing the ball, person to person, until everyone has had the ball once. Each person is to note whom they get the ball from and throw it to. The easiest way to track the creation of the pattern is for everyone to raise their hand, then lower it after they have caught the ball. The pattern begins and ends with the first ball thrower.

Once the pattern is established, have the group practice the pattern.

Next, start adding balls into the mix, coaching the players to continue throwing in the same pattern, all the while. It can be fun to surprise them with the increased complexity. You want at least three balls in play so the group is "juggling." The larger the group, the more balls you can add. (I have seen this game played with 50 people and 49 balls!)

How I Use This Game

This game illustrates Frank Pierce Jones's quote: "It was just as easy, I found, instead of setting up two fields—one for the self (introspection)

and one for the environment (extraspection)—to establish a single integrated field in which both the environment and the self could be viewed simultaneously" (Jones 1997, p.9).

I ask people, first, to focus on only the person they get it from and the person they throw it to. While the game works, it is often a bit choppy, and the longer it goes on, the more balls are dropped. Participants don't talk to each other or laugh much, being very much concerned about dropping the balls.

Then, I ask them to view the whole pattern rather than just focusing on the two people with whom they are directly involved. This might cause some initial ball dropping, but even if that happens at first, ultimately a more rhythmically regular pattern, smoother tosses, fewer ball drops, and a lot more fun, talking, and laughter usually ensue.

In addition, some people study the Alexander Technique to learn tools for stress management. (As previously noted, I think of stress as discoordinating while doing something that you want to do. You may have a lot to do, or not much time to do something, yet you still want to do it.) "Group Juggling" is a playful way to introduce "stress" into the classroom through the addition of more and more balls to the game. This offers players a chance to rehearse responding to what they consider to be stress by using Alexander Technique. I have also used this game when anyone's work and life involve many tasks as well as the need to switch these tasks constantly. In both these situations, adding more balls or complicating the task in other ways (such as providing a soundtrack of frantic classical music) can be helpful. It is easy and fun to create more variations.

The game is fun, creates an atmosphere of play and goodwill in the learning group, and can provide a needed change of pace in a longer workshop.

HAND SQUEEZE

Participants: At least 5

Source: Learned during my actor training

Description

Everyone stands in a circle holding hands. The teacher squeezes the hand of the person next to them, who, in turn, squeezes the hand of the person next to them, and so on around the circle. The idea is to pass the hand squeeze around the circle as fast as possible—which can be very rapid, indeed.

How I Use This Game

Creating and sending around a moving handshake makes a lovely closing game, a quick way for everyone to think their thank yous for the work we have done together.

HOP WHEN I SAY WALK

Participants: At least 2; more is better

Source: Adapted from a game I learned at an Association of Theatre Movement Educators Workshop

Description

In this game, familiar action words such as *walk*, *clap*, and *nod* are redefined, and then the group is asked to respond in action to the new definitions. For example, *walk* could mean hop, *clap* could mean turn in a circle, and *nod* might mean clap. To play the game, choose a leader. The Leader calls out "walk," "clap," or "nod" multiple times in a random order, then the group responds, using the new, redefined meanings. As you might imagine, hilarity often ensues as people play with the scrambled meanings.

The original words can be any words that define an action people can do; you can also have more than three, if you like. You can create many further variations, increasing complexity and interaction.

How I Use This Game

A learning cohort can learn to laugh amid the trials and errors of experimentation through games like this. It also offers an opportunity to use the Alexander Technique to choose how to respond to the words as they are called out.

HORSES AND RIDERS

Participants: 2 or more, done in pairs

Source: Learned from horseback riders I have taught

Description

Ask everyone to find a partner. Person A begins as the "horse," while Person B is the "rider." The rider stands behind the horse, putting their hands on the horse's torso. Using the Alexander Technique throughout, the rider experiments with different ways to ask the horse to go somewhere.

Options

A. The rider thinks where they want to go, looks where they want to go, and starts moving in that direction, noting how the horse responds (the horse, in this case, intends to cooperate).

B. The rider tells the horse via their hands where they want to go (the horse still intends to cooperate).

C. The rider uses option A, but the horse intends to be mischievous. When the horse starts off in another direction than the rider intends, the rider renews their option A plan.

D. Same as C, but the rider uses option B.

Many variations are possible.

How I Use This Game

This game is intended to give riders an idea of how different ways of tactile communication cause different responses in the horse. In our version, while it isn't a direct analogy to using your hands to teach the Alexander Technique, it is a playful way to experiment with using your hands in communication.

HUMAN PUZZLE

Participants: Ideally, 5 or more

Source: Adapted from *The New Games Book* (Fluegelman 1976, p.69)

Description

Everyone stands in a small circle, relatively close to each other. Give the preliminary instruction: "Reach across the circle to hold hands with two different people. Please don't cross your own arms." It sometimes takes a while to sort things out, and may involve some redoing as everyone manages to find two people. If any crossed arms ensue, more reorganizing becomes necessary. Now, give the main instruction: "Without letting go of each other's hands, please untangle." (People can, of course, change their grip if the angles get uncomfortable.) Amazingly, most of the time, the group manages to untangle and end up in a big circle together. Sometimes, a group ends up in two, or even three, intersecting circles.

How I Use This Game

Because this game requires using the Alexander Technique in multiple shapes and angles, it emphasizes that the Alexander Technique is about movement rather than posture. Usually this game is fun, but, occasionally, someone gets frustrated that the group is not solving the puzzle fast enough. This creates an opportunity to coach people to use the Alexander Technique when they are frustrated. Everyone has to work together to untangle, so the game is another way to build trust in a learning community.

INTEGRATIVE ALEXANDER TECHNIQUE ROUND ROBIN: VARIATION ONE (DAILY LIFE)

Participants: Groups of 3 to 20 are best; more are possible but will make the game lengthy

Supplies: Slips of paper; other props for the component activities can be useful but are not necessary

Source: Cathy Madden

Description

Note: This game takes a good bit of time. With a class of 16, it will take approximately an hour.

Before class, prepare slips of paper so there is one for everyone. Write various times of day on the papers, ranging from morning to night, so that the whole day is covered. Put the papers in a box or bowl.

Players pick a slip of paper out of the bowl, then arrange themselves in a circle that goes in time order from morning to night. They think of something that they might do at their time of day.

Begin with the person who has the earliest time, and use the chosen activity for that time as the activity for the lesson. Analyze, step by step, what needs to happen to do the activity, and use the Alexander Technique for each step. For instance, if the chosen activity is "turning off the alarm," the steps could be opening eyes, turning head to the left, rolling torso to the left, flexing the right elbow, extending the right elbow with fingers leading to the clock, fingers moving to quiet the alarm. Then, use the Alexander Technique for each step of the process. I usually pick one of the steps to examine in further detail.

What you might say to coach through the alarm clock activity:

- "Ask to COORDINATE so that your head can move so that all of you can follow so that you can open your eyes."

- "Ask to COORDINATE so that your head can move so that all of you can follow so that you can turn your head to the left."

- "Ask to COORDINATE so that your head can move so that all of you can follow so that you can roll your torso to the left."

- "Ask to COORDINATE so that your head can move so that all of you can follow so that you can flex your right elbow."

- "Ask to COORDINATE so that your head can move so that all of you can follow so that you can extend your right elbow with your fingers leading to the clock."

- "Ask to COORDINATE so that your head can move so that all of you can follow so that you can move your fingers to shut off the alarm."

Then, invite everyone to join in and do the whole sequence.

Now, go to the person who is next in the timeline. Repeat the process for the activity the person has selected for their time of day, including everyone doing it together at the end. Then, everyone does the first one, then the second one. Continue this way around the circle.

By the end, you are doing a sequence of Alexander Technique-infused activities that are part of daily life. Everyone has deeply investigated as many activities as there are people in the room, rehearsing them many times.

How I Use This Game

This game demonstrates how to integrate the Alexander Technique into many newly created studied rehearsed plans associated with daily life external cues—activities that are constantly practiced. For many students, this game has led to "Aha! Now I understand how to integrate the Alexander Technique into what I do."

INTEGRATIVE ALEXANDER TECHNIQUE ROUND ROBIN: VARIATION TWO (YOGA ASANA CREATION)

Participants: 3 to 20

Supplies: Whatever participants need for yoga

Source: Cathy Madden

Description

Same note as Variation One: This takes a long time, and it is a great integrative tool. This version originated in a Yoga and Alexander Technique workshop in Tokyo. Proceed just as in Variation One, but this time everyone chooses one yoga-related movement. As you go around the circle, the group gradually creates their own unique yoga asana.

How I Use This Game

Just as in Variation One, this game demonstrates how to integrate Alexander Technique while creating many studied rehearsed plans associated with yoga movement. It helps create some external cues to remember the Alexander Technique in any yoga pose. Because the group creates something unique to them, the game builds the learning cohort.

INTEGRATIVE ALEXANDER TECHNIQUE ROUND ROBIN: VARIATION THREE (MORE ACTIVITIES)

Participants: 3 to 20

Supplies: Whatever participants desire for their chosen task

Source: Cathy Madden

Description

Again, this takes a long time, and it is a great integrative tool.

The instructions are the same as Variation Two. The activities, however, could be selected from any field. If you are teaching a group of runners, you could use this game to create a warm-up for running with person-by-person contributions. (You can monitor the choices for health.) A group of musicians might create a short composition. Dancers might create a dance or a warm-up. Artists could create a drawing. Computer programmers might create code. Dog walkers could create all kinds of imaginary scenarios of what might happen and what they might need to do while taking a dog for a walk. The options are endless.

How I Use This Game

Just as in the other variations, this game demonstrates how to integrate the Alexander Technique while creating many studied rehearsed plans associated with activities associated with a specific skill set. It is both a creative process and a cohort-building process.

MAKE A SPINE

Participants: Larger group of at least 10

Source: Cathy Madden

Description

The group stands and decides a giant person is lying on the floor, looking out the window, head at one end of the room and feet at another. Then, they become the spine of the giant by standing in the shape of the spine, putting their hands on the mid-torso of the person in front of them, the hands representing the intervertebral disks. At this point, a bit of mayhem ensues as people work on this. Often, the first iteration leaves out the spinal curves; then, the group has to work together to figure out where the curves are. Once we have a fairly reasonable looking imaginary spine, the game is over.

Variation

Use this spinal sculpture to illustrate "all of you can follow." The teacher becomes the head and pushes down on the top of the spine, first asking the person at the end to stay in place and reminding everyone else they can move their feet. This demonstrates that, when you put pressure in the system, everything gets squished. Now, reverse it by "using the Alexander Technique" on this imaginary spine, with the head moving, all the vertebrae following.

How I Use This Game

This is a playful way to review anatomy and demonstrate what I mean by "all of you can follow."

MUSICAL CHAIRS (ALEXANDER TECHNIQUE STYLE)

Participants: Best with 5 or more

Supplies: Chairs, all different kinds, one fewer than the number of participants

Source: Adapted from my childhood

Description

In a workshop, one of the participants was asking about how to deal with all kinds of chairs—talking in a way that made her sound as if the chair were in charge of her coordination. I remembered assisting Marj at a workshop, in which the chairs were particularly poorly designed. She was teaching small groups sequentially, and each time a new group came in, they would complain about the chairs. As one group arrived, they saw Marj touching one of the chairs, moving her hands to different spots on the chair and waiting, then moving her hands somewhere else. Everyone watched, unsure what she was up to, until she said, "It won't change." She had been giving the chair an Alexander Technique lesson to no avail! There was no more complaining about the chairs.

As I thought about this incident with Marj along with my student's question, I wanted to find a playful way to put her in charge of the chairs. At break time, I went around my house and brought a multitude of different kinds of chairs to my studio. Everyone had a turn using Alexander Technique to sit in each chair, analyzing the physics, anatomy, and geometry required, then creating appropriate plans for each one.

Once we had studied rehearsed plans for each chair, we played musical chairs: everyone walks around the chairs while music is playing, and when the music stops, everyone scrambles for the nearest chair. Repeat, removing a chair after each round; with one fewer chair available, not everyone gets to sit down. The larger idea is that we have created a variety of Alexander Technique-based plans for sitting, which we are now using at the speed of daily life.

How I Use This Game

The impetus to create this game was primarily to playfully illustrate that we have a choice about how we sit in chairs. The chairs have no choice.

It is a playful way to examine the anatomy, physics, and geometry of an action we do every day. Because everyone is a different size in relationship to each kind of chair, everyone gets to experience how omniservation is important. The repetition of the same essential action—sitting—offers the possibility for guiding everyone to omniserve with greater detail in each repetition. From this omniservation, they learn how to build a detailed, constructive plan.

As with many of the games, the competition and speed factors enable people to practice responding to daily life demands by coordinating rather than tightening.

NAME AND MOVEMENT CIRCLE

Participants: Best with 5 or more

Source: Adapted from multiple sources

Description

Everyone stands in a circle, and I ask them to make a movement as they say their name. I first demonstrate using a gesture that is in three planes of movement and at least medium-sized, hoping to allay any shyness in the group. I ask everyone to remember the movement they chose. After our first round of movements and names, I ask everyone to "scrunch" a little between head and spine and do the same thing again. We immediately get to see and hear the effects of the compromised head–spine relationship. If you use this game to help introduce the Alexander Technique, this provides a moment for a bit of background information about F.M. Alexander's discovery. Then, I ask the group to do it one more time, this time starting "scrunched" and using the Alexander Technique partway through the movement to restore their coordination while moving.

How I Use This Game

This is sometimes a second-night game in a new Alexander Technique class. People are still learning names, and often a few people will have joined the class late and missed the introduction. This game helps new people to catch up with the information from the first night and, while not an exact repeat, serves as a useful refresher for everyone. My emphasis is on the practicality of using Alexander Technique while you are doing something—from the beginning.

ONE, TWO, THREE

Participants: At least 2

Source: Adapted from "Two by Three by Bradford" in *Games for Actors and Non-Actors* (Boal 2002[1992], p.106)

Description
First Set-Up

Two people stand opposite each other. Person A, who always starts the sequence, says, "One." Person B says, "Two." Person A says, "Three." Then, Person B returns to, "One," Person A says, "Two," Person B says, "Three," and you're back around to Person A saying, "One." Keep doing this until you see that everyone, or most everyone, has had a good laugh. It seems like an easy game, but becomes strangely difficult as you do it over and over.

Second Set-Up

Game play is the same, with one exception: instead of saying, "One," Person A makes a movement (a) that replaces saying the word. The sequence then repeats movement (a), "Two," "Three," movement (a), "Two," "Three." Again, play until the room is laughing, at least a little.

Third Set-Up

Now, Person B makes up a movement (b) to replace saying, "Two." The alternating sequence becomes movement (a), movement (b), "Three."

Fourth Set-Up

As you have probably guessed, this is the all-movement version of the game. Person A replaces saying, "Three," with making movement (c). Now, the alternating sequence is solely movement: (a), (b), (c).

How I Use This Game

Since partners are looking at each other, they are practicing omniservational skills.

This game fools you—it seems like it should be quite simple. Every group I have taught it to has been surprised by the mistakes that creep in. The mistakes are fun and funny, a whimsical reminder that we always have something we can learn. The group of partners tends to become one learning cohort, experiencing errors in a safe way.

In an experienced group, this game offers practice in responding to perceived adversity by asking to COORDINATE rather than compromising the head–spine relationship. The game setting facilitates experimentation—because there are no direct consequences in the outside world.

PAPER PEOPLE

Participants: Any number

Supplies: A piece of paper for everyone—I like to give legal-sized (or larger) sheets, and colored paper is even more fun; crayons or colored markers are optional, when time permits

Source: Adapted from a workshop with Jean Illsley Clarke

Description

I often offer this game in the first class, as people are arriving. Everyone receives a sheet of paper with the instruction "Please tear a person out of the sheet of paper." If they ask for further instructions, I just say the same words again. Usually, I am also doing the activity, so they have a moving/visual version of the instruction to model as well.

The cohort of paper people has a variety of uses. Sometimes, I ask people to write a note about why they are taking the class on the back.

Sometimes, I ask them to put their name on the front and it becomes their class nametag. Often, I use picking these paper people off the floor as the first experiment in using the Alexander Technique.

If I am doing a longer workshop, I might give everyone crayons to color their paper people. I have learned to do this only for a several-day workshop because adults seem to be coloring-deprived and can spend 45 minutes or more coloring their paper people.

How I Use This Game

The Paper People game is a gentle signal that this class is going to be unusual. It is impossible to tear out paper people right or wrong. A few people try to regularize their work by folding the paper in half so the two sides of their person are symmetrical (which offers me potential information about how they learn)—but the edges are always ragged.

Sometimes, the Paper People shapes offer clues about someone's idea of themselves. A violinist laughed, realizing the paper puppet he had made had arms that lifted forward in violin-holding shape; an extremely tall women (who had been given a legal size sheet of paper) tore out a figure one inch tall; some are missing parts. They aren't Rorschach tests, yet they may proffer clues I'll need as I teach the class.

While you could play this game at any time, I usually use it before the first class. It gives people something to do while others are arriving, while facilitating casual chatter. Everyone, after all, is in the same situation—adults asked to do crafts at the start of a coordination class.

PIPE CLEANER CREATIONS (AND OTHER TOYS FOR TEACHING)

Description

This is a varied section for toys that might be useful in teaching. They are games with a slightly different slant.

Pipe Cleaner Collection

My student and colleague, Ken Anno, embraced the spirit of deep play in my studio some years ago, creating myriad pipe cleaner creatures of dazzling variety, including some that are useful for teaching. His pipe cleaner skeletons are marvels of specificity, even fashioned so as to show movement. He created the aforementioned turquoise spotted platypus to illustrate what to think of when you don't want to think about a pink elephant. I also have a collection of pipe cleaner chickens that I can distribute as needed per "Finger Puppet Monsters and Rubber Chickens." His handmade creations spark wonder in all.

Handmade items are an added bonus when you are lucky enough to have them, or, in the case of my pipe cleaner set, to be gifted with them. Even a small handmade touch on a hand-out serves the learning relationship. Your students recognize another way in which you have invested in them.

Pea Shooters

For this game, I give each of my workshop members a pea shooter with paper balls. Everyone "shoots" off a paper ball each time they learn something new. Offering a way to, in essence, "shout" that you have learned something emphasizes the joy of new learning. Using the pea shooter to celebrate learning also keeps the group on its toes— you never know when one is coming!

Wish Capsules

These miniature pill-sized capsules contain a piece of paper, on which students can write their wish for a workshop. It is a lovely, quiet way for a group that is new to one another to do something unusual together that wakes up their desire to be there, but it is also private.

Plastic Pink Elephant

"Don't" messages run rampant in many of our biopsychosocial histories. In some workshops, we play with giving someone a small plastic pink elephant whenever we hear a "don't" statement.

Slinky

The Slinky can be a fun way to explain how the head moves and all of you follows. I have a moon-shaped Slinky that looks almost like a vertebra. They can be great for explaining the Alexander Technique to kids.

Blank Dice

At a workshop in Munich, my host Gudrun Lehn gave everyone a blank die. As I saw them, I thought, "This would be a great way for someone to say they are ready for a turn; they just roll the dice. The blank sides serve as a reminder that we are moving into the unknown and have no idea what will happen."

The Friday Harbor Residential

My annual residential includes a feast of toys. I supply at least one new toy per day, attempting to match them to whatever the year's theme is. As the workshop is held on a marine preserve, we are often sea creature-themed, though recently our theme was river otters. The presence of so many toys nurtures an ongoing expectation of play; it gives full, deep permission for adults to enjoy, for example throwing glow-in-the-dark sea stars in a night-time version of group juggling.

PRUI

Participants: Best with 5 or more

Source: Adapted from *The New Games Book* (Fluegelman 1976, p.133)

Description

Tell everyone that, in a moment, you will ask the group to close their eyes, then you'll touch someone to indicate the person who will become Prui. Once Prui is selected, everyone—still with their eyes closed—will search for Prui. Remind everyone that you have your eyes open to keep them safe. (If it is a large room with many players, then you may want to recruit several other people to help with this.) I walk around the room several times, talking all the while as I designate Prui, hoping to disguise whom I pick. Once you have made your selection, invite people to start walking—and, yes, they will bump into each other.

When a person runs into someone, they say, "Prui." If the person bumped into responds, "Prui," then they know they have not found Prui and move on. If they run into someone who does not answer, then they know by Prui's silence that they have found Prui. Once a person has found Prui, they also become Prui, remain attached to whomever they ran into, and are silent when someone runs into them as well. Eventually, everyone finds Prui, which is now a silent clump of people.

How I Use This Game

Because players' eyes are closed, this game heightens nonvisual omniservation skills. I have used it to remind people that we orient to sound as well as sight.

When a group has been working intensely and needs a break, this game is great fun!

RENAME THAT OBJECT

Participants: Any number

Source: Judy Shahn, a colleague at the University of Washington, taught me this game

Description

Players walk around the room, pointing at various objects, shouting out a new name for each object. The aim is to rename loudly everything they see. For example, pointing at a chair and shouting, "Hairbrush!" After a few minutes of this, the group pauses, and for most people, the room looks different simply because of all the names that are changed.

How I Use This Game

Teaching and learning the Alexander Technique requires flexibility in sorting through your perceptions. This game reveals how quickly something as simple as changing the names of things alters your perception of the space around you. Because it is quick and loud, it can be a good mood-shifter in a longer workshop. It also jostles familiar thinking patterns in a playful way. Sometimes, this game can help people accept my "invented verb" practice.

SCULPTURE OMNISERVATION

Participants: At least 4; more is better

Source: Cathy Madden

Description

Half of the participants form Group A, while the others are Group B. (In very large groups, you could create more than two small groups.) Group A faces away from Group B, while Group B together create a human sculpture. When Group B is ready, they ask Group A to turn around and admire their creation. After one minute, the teacher asks Group B to dissolve their sculpture, then asks Group A to recreate the sculpture they just saw. (Ideally this is a surprise.) When Group A thinks they have finished making their sculpture, Group B adjusts anything that needs adjusting.

Then you reverse the tasks. This time, however, since Group B knows what they will be asked to do, give them 45 seconds rather than a full minute.

Play as many times as you like.

How I Use This Game

This game primarily exercises omniservation skills, but it is also a fun, active game if you need a change of pace. The learning cohort works together toward a goal, often accompanied by laughter.

SIX-ASPECT CREATURE

Participants: 6 to many

Source: Cathy Madden

Description

Ask everyone to get into groups of six. Within these groups of six, players make a sculpture of some sort so that everyone is in contact, touching at least two other people. The sculpture is ideally relatively simple, because they will be staying in it for a while.

Each group of six metaphorically becomes one creature with six aspects. Each person in a creature is assigned an aspect of humanness: physical, mental, emotional, spiritual, social, and mystery. While I offer the spiritual possibility, I note that if this is not an aspect someone has in their conception of wholeness, then they are exempt from taking on that role. I include the mystery aspect because I don't want to assume that we know all there is to know about being human. Hence, Six-Aspect Creature.

I continue by finding someone from the whole group who wants a turn. They leave their creature, and we adjust the roles in that particular small group.

During the turn, if an aspect seems to relate to the lesson I am teaching, the person in each group representing that aspect moves. Which means everyone in the creature moves. Every aspect moves when the lesson includes it, which means that, often, more than one person is actively moving. Because everyone passively moves with each active movement, the small groups start undulating. This continual movement of all the creatures is a visible representation of wholeness of self.

Do this for at least five individual lessons, with people switching the aspect they represent each time until everyone actively experiences each aspect.

How I Use This Game

This game teaches wholeness of self while serving as an active omniservation game. I created it for a workshop in Osaka, when people kept asking me what I meant by "whole self."

THIS IS MY NOSE

Participants: 2 or more, done in pairs

Source: Adapted from *More New Games* (Fluegelman 1981, p.27)

Description

Two people face each other. One person points to a body part, for example, their knee, and calls it anything other than a knee—for instance, a nose. Their partner then points to the part the first player named—in this case, the nose—and names it anything other than a nose. The conversation sounds and moves like this:

"This is my nose" (while pointing to the knee)

"This is my knee" (while pointing to the elbow)

"This is my elbow" (while pointing to the right foot)

"This is my right foot" (while pointing to the ear)

Continue as long as desired.

How I Use This Game

This game is a playful way to begin an anatomy session, bring a session to a close, or both. Sometimes, I use it to begin class the day after an anatomy session as an entertaining review/renewal of the previous material. I once taught this to a group who had an anatomy exam the next day, and they got extremely detailed—it turned out to be an excellent study tool.

The larger point of the game is that it is "right" to say the "wrong" thing. For students whose previous education has been inextricably bound to being right, this game can be a challenge—which turns into a lot of laughter. The game also creates moments of fun in relationship with a partner, so it functions well as a learning community builder.

WALK, CLAP, NOD

Participants: At least 6

Source: Learned in a eurhythmy class

Description

The group stands in a circle. Everyone learns a pattern that moves into the center of the circle and backs out. The pattern is walk in three steps, clap three times, nod three times. This is followed by walk out three steps, clap three times, nod three times. The rhythm of the pattern is one beat per word: walk, walk, walk, clap, clap, clap, nod, nod, nod.

After everyone practices the pattern a few times—going into the center and backing out on the walks—ask the group to count off by twos. Play the game again, but, this time, in a kind of musical round: The 1s start, then the 2s start while the 1s move on to clapping.

The pattern is shown in Table 29.1.

Table 29.1 Walk, Clap, Nod Pattern

1s	2s
walk (in)	
walk	
walk	
clap	walk (in)
clap	walk
clap	walk
nod	clap
nod	clap
nod	clap
walk (out)	nod
walk	nod
walk	nod
clap	walk(out)
clap	walk
clap	walk

...and so on.

Variation One

With a larger group, you can have three groups moving as in a three-part musical round.

Variation Two

Coach everyone to walk anywhere rather than in and out of the circle. After they have moved away from each other, still using the pattern, invite them to return to their original placement.

How I Use This Game

In addition to practice using the Alexander Technique for three daily life tasks—walking, clapping, nodding—this game demonstrates the importance and effectiveness of staying with each task as it happens.

WHOLE GROUP MOVING OMNISERVATION

Participants: At least 4, best with 8 or more

Source: I learned it in a workshop

Description

Ask the whole group to get up and start walking around the room. Then ask each person to secretly pick one other person to keep in their field of attention—ideally, in their visual field as well. Everyone keeps walking as they endeavor to keep their chosen person secretly in their attention. Once the group has done this for a while, while everyone is still walking (no pause in this game), ask everyone to pick a second secret person, then keep both secret partners in their attention while continuing to walk around the room.

Again, after a few minutes, ask everyone to continue moving until they form an equilateral triangle with their two secret partners. As they arrive in the equilateral triangle, they stop moving. Often, this takes many times as the group picture keeps moving and shifting. If a group has a perfectionist in it, you may need to coach them to form "roughly" equilateral triangles or it may take longer than you wish to come to stillness.

How I Use This Game

This game is useful for omniservation practice, experiments with peripersonal and extrapersonal space, group interaction, and a bit of beauty—the patterns that emerge when everyone comes to stillness can be quite lovely.

WHOLENESS DANCE

Participants: 1 to 500

Source: Cathy Madden (Madden 2014, pp.350–351)

Description

If someone says something that contains a mind/body split, or is somehow divisive of self, anyone can call for the wholeness dance. The sequence of the dance:

> Front Side, Back Side
> Right Side, Left Side
> Up Side, Down Side
> Inside, Outside
> All Sides, Always!

For each side, the Leader (usually the teacher) says—for example—"front side" while doing a gesture or movement to that side; then the group repeats the Leader's words and movement. You do this for each of the "sides" until you gleefully reach "all sides, always"—for your final movement, dancing in a circle with your fingers wiggling in the air.

How I Use This Game

I use this game to emphasize our wholeness in a playful group-inclusive way. People sometimes do it for themselves when they can't think of a way to say something "whole" but do intend to mean "whole self." I give the group permission to call for this dance anytime.

YAMANOTE LINE

Participants: 1 or more

Supplies: This game is suitable in any city that has a mass transit circular line, for example, Tokyo, Seoul, London, or Moscow

Source: Cathy Madden

Description

I created a game in Tokyo, involving a metaphor between the AT Progression and the Yamanote line, a train line that makes a circular route around Tokyo. The game resonates best with a group if the city you are in has a circular train line. (It would not work well in Seattle, for example, where the light rail runs roughly in a straight line. We could create a fictional train line, but there is something energizing about the biopsychosocial response when the participants regularly ride a circular line.)

Create AT Progression stations in a circle around a central area where turns occur. The rest of the group travels station to station, AT Progression stop to AT Progression stop, going to the station they think corresponds to the lesson. As with the Yamanote and other circular lines, the train doesn't go backward to a stop, it always moves forward.

How I Use This Game

People learn the AT Progression more as they move with it. I created it specially to show that, although the steps in the AT Progression repeat, we are not reverting to a former step, but rather always moving forward into the next iteration of that step.

Chapter 30

TIPS FOR TURNS

Having traversed Alexander Technique teaching skills, perspectives from research in adult learning and human expertise, discussions of a variety of teaching structures, and even a few games, we reach the juncture F.M. Alexander described in *The Use of the Self*:

> It is impossible in the space at my command to put down all the details of the variations of the teacher's art that were employed to bring my pupil to this point, for a teacher's technique naturally varies in detail according to the particular needs and difficulties of each pupil. (Alexander 1984[1932], p.73)

This chapter, then, comprises a selection of short vignettes, alphabetically organized, in which I share a few ideas that have proved helpful to me over the years as I've negotiated the Alexander Technique teaching variations.

All of You Follows

A longtime student asked, "What does 'so that all of you can follow' really mean?"

I was puzzled. For me, it seems quite simple. When you move one end of a string, the rest simply follows. When you tie your shoe, the lace moves—follows—in the way your hand leads. Your hand moves and the lace follows. If children all hold hands in a line, then the child at the head of the line starts to walk, all the children follow. The "all," in the case of a person, is more biopsychosocially complex than a string, so how the follow manifests is unpredictable; yet, it is as simple in process as leader–follower.

Our class that day began outdoors. As we gathered to go inside, it occurred to me that I was leading and everyone else was following. My walk was a beeline from my spot on the bluff to the door of the lecture hall. Others collected their bags, picked up their cups, even rounded up a toddler. Everyone took a slightly different trajectory to "follow." All individual. All achieved the desired outcome. I moved, everyone followed, in their unique, necessary, perfect way. Once inside, we drew a map of all of our trajectories so we could picture the phrase "all of you can follow" as an invitation with many variations of response.

Anatomy

A student got a lot of notes about his hips. When I started talking about his hips, he ranted, "What does everyone mean? I keep thinking about them and nothing happens." I said, "Forget about your hips! Let's see what happens if you start to move at the joint between your leg and your pelvis." Suddenly, his movement was pristine.

Another time, a student suddenly asked, "Cathy, what do you mean by torso?" I explained that I meant everything from the occiput to the joint between the leg and pelvis. He said, "You don't mean a little circle here?" while pointing at a spot just below the xiphoid process. In that moment, he updated his definition of *torso* (a word I now use carefully) and was much more effective when he asked himself to COORDINATE! We imagined that, perhaps when he was a child, he had a beginning anatomy book—and the line from the word *torso* ended at that spot.

Recently, at a large lecture, someone asked about breathing. Because of how she described breathing, I was fairly certain she thought her lungs were in her belly. I asked everyone to point to where their lungs were, and most pointed too low. I showed everyone where the lungs actually are, and I wish I had a video to show how everyone in the room was immediately moving better.

Anatomy matters because how we think we are made manifests in our behavior. I taught the Alexander Technique effectively when I knew less anatomy than I know now; each new bit of knowledge augments my effectiveness.

The Art of the Handout

Some students like handouts. I never particularly needed written material when I studied the Alexander Technique. However, I learned that some people learn better with visible structure. One way I can take care of them is by offering handouts.

My choices regarding handouts reflect my predilection for play. At an International Congress of the Alexander Technique in Lugano, I handwrote the handouts on lace doilies—since I was introducing the idea of "invite." For a workshop for harpists, I put all the text into the shape of a harp, and once printed, cut the harps out of the paper. At the very least, I use festive paper and, like the teachers in a Waldorf school, cut the corners of the paper into rounded edges to create a more moving, organic shape. In my studio, I offer simple handouts, preprinted on colorful postcards, with key phrases that I use in teaching.

Handmade is a value for me, particularly with new groups. And when I can, I like to offer the sheet to each student personally. Both of these gestures convey the message that I am personally invested in their learning. Offering the handout as a gift invites participation; receiving it may be the first "yes" of the lesson.

Belief Changers

Most of Alexander Technique teaching develops new beliefs. I use *belief changer* specifically to describe moments in lessons when I make up something—either a movement or an activity—to help someone get the information they need to change an idea.

It is one of the things I did for myself as I was learning. For example, when I realized that I was tightening my arms in a particular way to go up the stairs, and despite a variety of Alexander Technique experiments was still behaving as if my arms could move my legs, I fashioned another test. I stood in front of the stairs and made only the arm movement—to see if that would get me up the stairs. Of course, it was a bit silly because I knew it wouldn't work. Yet, this really helped me make the desired change in my pattern. I had to prove it to myself in action.

A violinist who seemed not to believe that he could bend his left elbow provides a teaching example. His left arm was stuck at one slightly bent angle in the violin-holding shape. Showing him anatomy images didn't help. He was using the Alexander Technique, but he was using it to hold his arm in that particular shape. I finally was able to challenge his belief when I found a soft sweater. I put it in his left hand, noting that it was soft. The tone in his arm muscles changed slightly, and I quickly moved his left lower arm so that it was now bent enough that he could touch his shoulder blade. He was surprised.

Belief changers are one-time events. They are meant to biopsychosocially challenge an outdated idea.

Big Picture, Little Picture

In the workshop that I took with Jean Illsley Clarke, I reconsidered the organization of teaching. I had always been puzzled by a few learners who seemed to have a very hard time with information that others picked up easily. I knew that they needed something different from what I was offering, and that this something had to do with structure. In her book, *Who, Me Lead a Group?*, Clarke describes two primary ways adult learners like to organize their learning:

> Adults organize new information as they collect it, but not all of them organize it in the same way. Some of them prefer to get an overview of the material—a big picture—or an abstract theory, and then see where various parts of the concrete experiences fit in. Other adults organize learning material by searching about for bits and pieces, or even large chunks, from which to create their own view of the big picture. (Clarke 1984, p.21)

She continues:

> The people who need the big picture first are very goal-oriented. They are uncomfortable when asked to do something unless there is an explanation first indicating how the activity contributes to their larger goal. (Clarke 1984, p.21)

I learned to start a workshop in a way that said, "I have a larger picture, and each thing along the way will contribute to it." Sometimes, I am explicit about the larger picture; sometimes, I am not, because being explicit would compromise a step-by-step approach. In the latter case, however, I can tell the big-picture people that the goal is to learn a step-by-step approach.

Celebrating Success

As a teacher, recognizing success so that the student credits themselves for their work is key to their ownership of the work. And the only one who can actually do the work that creates success in an Alexander Technique lesson is the student. Teachers can acknowledge success verbally, and I also have a few ways to encourage students to congratulate themselves.

In one workshop I attended (not on the Alexander Technique), the leader handed out letter-size cardstock with an odd cut creating a funny-shaped hole in our cardboard. She asked us to hold up the paper in front of our face, then look at the world through that shape. Her analogy was that, with our current information, we saw the world through this limited lens. She invited us to tear out a bit more of the paper—widening the shape—each time, we learned something. At the end of the workshop, we looked at each other through our expanded worldview.

In longer-range workshops, I also like to give people a way to "mark" their success—sometimes, with a toy they can throw in the air or a kazoo they can play. Perhaps there is a group bulletin board on which everyone can "draw" their success in some way, or a journal you give them specifically for celebration purpose.

Or, it might simply be a momentary personal dance of joy shared with the group.

Chemical Baths

This title comes from a slightly humorous interpretation of Candace Pert's *Molecules of Emotion*, regarding how emotion and memory may be stored chemically in a variety of places, including contracted muscle. "If we accept the idea that peptides and other informational substances are the biochemicals of emotion, their distribution in the body's nerves has all kinds of significance... The body is the unconscious mind" (Pert 1997, p.141). Sometimes, in an Alexander Technique lesson, someone starts to cry; sometimes, they don't even feel sad, but suddenly they are crying. What is going on?

This happened to me, in fact, at one of Marj's Nebraska workshops. I had learned something about sound making during the morning workshop, discovering something about the back of my mouth.

What became somewhat funny that day was that, unless I was teaching, I had to cry or yawn or go back to my old pattern. I chose to alternate between crying and yawning because my sound was so much better without the old pattern. When I got tired of one, I'd do the other. I didn't feel sad, but I suspect some "molecules of emotion" associated with unexpressed sadness in the past had been released, causing the need to cry. Because I wanted to continue the change I had made, I cried or yawned until the need for that disappeared.

Occasionally, a student goes through a spell of tears coming at every lesson. And many of them really don't like it. I've taken to calling these events "chemical baths" as a way of making them okay, even a little humorous.

Humor

In *Direction* magazine's issue spotlighting Marjorie Barstow, there is a wonderful picture of her wearing a rather outlandish hat and her cauliflower T-shirt with the quote "Learn to laugh at yourselves: you always move better with a smile" (Barstow and Brenner 1987, p.37).

Perhaps that is the best place to begin this discussion—before you use humor in teaching, you need to be willing to laugh at yourself, too.

When I think of humor, I always turn to a gem of a book, *The Craft of Comedy* by Athene Seyler and Stephen Haggard. Seyler's advice holds for teaching with humor:

> Comedy, shall I say, is the sparkle on the water, not the depths beneath; the gay surface, the glint of sunlight—any other pretty metaphor. But note, the waters must run deep underneath. In other words, comedy must be founded on truth and on an understanding of a real value of a character before it can pick out the high-lights. It is only when one thoroughly understands a person that one can afford to laugh at him.
>
> And here I would stipulate another quality that I find indispensable to the comic spirit—that of good nature. I am aware that this is a debatable point and that it may well be a personal idiosyncrasy of my own, but to me comedy is inextricably bound up with kindliness. (Seyler and Haggard 1946, p.11)

I share Seyler's idiosyncrasy. Humor in teaching has its roots in honesty and kindness.

If You Think You Need to Refer It to Another Professional, You Do

The Alexander Technique doesn't do everything. It just doesn't.

It is a lovely "how" that restores what is restorable so it can serve you well.

If the student's question or need involves something broken, or out of place, in any of the biopsychosocial spheres, you might find yourself stumped or frightened.

This has happened a few times in my teaching career—not many, but a few. I referred them to medical care.

It is rare that I won't teach someone until they seek the other help, but it has happened a few times. And I have been glad each time I made this choice.

It Isn't Always Use

With some activities, the Alexander Technique helps me omniserve that the reason the student is not finding success in their task is not actually about coordination. They are, at least partially, experiencing difficulty for other reasons. I mentioned that I have hula hoops in my studio. They are there not because I think everyone needs to hula hoop, but because they are a reminder that not all solutions involve the Alexander Technique. The inspiration for this was when someone was trying to learn to hula hoop using the Alexander Technique, and it didn't "work" until they discovered that adults need adult-sized hula hoops for the physics to work.

Another student wanted to work on her "high notes" in singing. I had to convince her to sing some scales first—all the Alexander Technique in the world was not going to help her sing a high note unless she warmed up her resonators by making sound. The Alexander Technique is good, but it doesn't defy the physics of sound.

One instrumentalist gave me some great feedback about teaching musicians that is related to this. She complained that, while she always felt better playing in her lessons, she wasn't convinced to value the technique because the tone of her instrument wasn't as good as she knew it could be. Physics!—the violin needed to be played a bit before it would ring optimally. I sent her off to warm herself and the instrument up before her turn. The results were more rewarding—she felt better and the tone was better, too!

Learning Something New Yourself

Finding opportunities to be a student (rather than a teacher) renews my appreciation of the hopefulness of our choice to learn or do something new. It reminds me that trust is earned by action. While I welcome walking the unknown as a teacher, as a student who doesn't know what to do or even what information to ask, walking the unknown is a different experience. The last "new" thing I did was to take an art class in charcoal portraiture. The joy of succeeding in learning new skills, capped by my teacher's celebration of my portrait of my grandfather, served notice that ongoing learning is vivifying and acknowledging student success is essential.

The Magic Is in Your Coordination

Sometimes, people ascribe magic to the Alexander Technique, perhaps describing the teacher as magical. This can be an awkward moment. Clearly, the new information has had a significant welcome result. I honor their response, respect the joy of the new information, and then frame it in a way that gives the student ownership of the process. My back-pocket plan for this moment is to use the Alexander Technique to invite my students to be with me while I am with them as I say, "I think the magic is in how well we are designed. When we use this process, we rediscover our own magic." Marj sometimes said, "The 'magic,' if you want to call it magic, is in your constructive thinking" (Barstow and Brenner 1987, p.33).

Never Mind about That...

This phrase appeared at specific moments in my studies with Marj. She seemed to use it when someone had thoroughly analyzed a particular response/behavior and (my interpretation) Marj believed they could solve the problem they were posing themselves. Once I was doing a monologue—Hermia from *A Midsummer Night's Dream*:

Puppet? why so? ay, that way goes the game.
Now I perceive that she hath made compare
Between our statures; she hath urged her height;
And with her personage, her tall personage,
Her height, forsooth, she hath prevail'd with him.

(Shakespeare 1974, III, ii, 289–294, p.216)

As I described to Marj how I was interfering with my ability to do the acting—worried about not being loud enough, not being excited enough, not being funny—all things I had worked through before, she just stopped me, suggested, "never mind about all that, use the Alexander Technique and do what you know how to do." It worked very well—my friends were surprised at the sound that emerged!

I use "never mind about that" when I am teaching in the same kind of situation. The phrase doesn't help when students haven't done the homework to address what is going on. But, when they have, it reminds them to use a bit of "will" to do what they already know how to do.

Perfect

A key in my teaching and an idea deeply infused in my training is that we do everything perfectly based on our current information. A longtime student told me a story that apparently comes from the U.S. Forest Service: When the Forest Service decided to implement changes in forest management, the director was told that many of the people who had worked for the Forest Service for many years were highly upset. As he thought about it, he realized that the changes were making people who cared deeply about the forests think they had been wrong for what they had previously been doing. He convened regional meetings across the country to deliver the message: "We have been practicing state-of-the-art forestry throughout our history. The state of the art has changed. What remains the same is our commitment to state-of-the-art forestry." He framed the changes as perfect-to-perfect—which is the truth in our learning as well.

Taking Care of the Fear

Sometimes, trying out a new idea in coordination—either explicably or inexplicably—causes fear. What I have learned to do first is to assure and reassert safety in the place we are in at the present moment. It is often as simple as "Look around and see where you are, and see that you are, in every way we can assure it, safe." If you are teaching a group, then these moments usually prompt everyone to offer assurance to the student who is frightened.

I ask, is it a specific fear?

If it is specific, then the student and I begin a gentle bit of detection work to see how the Alexander Technique can respond to what has been revealed. It is not uncommon for this to relate to old accidents. One student discovered that her stiffening was a constant "keeping of herself from flying backward on her head" because she had been in an accident as a child. To take care of her fear, she needed to assess the situation and realize that she was in charge of her locomotion.

Some car accident victims are protecting themselves particularly in the direction of the impact of their event; for them, looking around in the studio and seeing that there are no cars about is the first step to sustaining their coordination. The next step is figuring out what plan they need when they are driving.

If the fear is general, looking around to see that they are safe may be all they need. They may still feel frightened. It is important to let fear be okay: "You can ask to COORDINATE so that your head can move so that all of you can follow so that you can know that you feel frightened and know you are safe at the same time." I may ask again, "What do you think you need to do to take care of the fear?"

While writing this, I thought of the children's song, "We're Going on a Bear Hunt," in which the protagonist keeps running into scary obstacles, responding that they "got to go through it!" (Rosen and Oxenbury 1989, pp.6–7).

Avoiding fear, or judging it wrong in some way, or disguising it, simply causes more tightening between head and spine. The Alexander Technique has revealed something that needs care. How do we care for the fear?

Sidere

A performer came into the studio and said she was terrified to sing a high note. Once again, I found myself confronted with an insistence on associating art and fear.

What I usually have done with this is to point out that doing something on the edge of a person's skill level does require a heightened state, which may be physiologically similar to fear. But really, it isn't the same—because it is something one wants.

Simply reframing fear as readiness wasn't working for this student; I wondered how I could be more specific—for her, and ultimately for others. We are talking about a specific state of being that includes excitation, which is why it gets confused as fear. Calling it fear, however, puts it in the same category as being chased by a wild animal or being exiled from your tribe. Singing a high note—or any act of learning something new—doesn't belong in that category. It is a sought out, deliberately chosen state of being originating from something we care about in our life or work.

As an already experienced neologist, I sought a new word. Since desire is a key element of these chosen experiences, my search landed on the root word of desire: sidere, or "from the stars." I loved the poetry of this derivation, which matches my belief that this artistic state of conscious engagement with the unknown for learning, creativity, exploration, and experimentation is magic, perhaps "from the stars."

I have been using this word for a few months now, and it has been effective. We now have a name for this state of being, enabling the student to be appropriately excited—and no longer afraid.

Teeth

In my undergraduate class at the University of Washington, I gave an assignment to apply the Alexander Technique to something you do every day. One student chose brushing her teeth. Apparently, she brushed her teeth in the living room of her apartment. Her roommates were curious about what she was doing, so she explained the assignment to them. Everyone in her household started experimenting with using the Alexander Technique to brush their teeth. The way she recounted the scene sounded like they were all having a lot of fun with it. The student reported that everyone in the apartment had improved the quality of their tooth brushing, though I had taught only her.

The Ten-Minute "Rule"

You never call anything in an Alexander Technique class a "rule"—our freedom to choose is so central to what we do. I do sometimes request, however, that a student wait ten minutes before asking questions after a particularly significant learning experience. My hope is to keep them with their newly discovered success for some moments before questioning it. Sometimes, at moments of big shifts, our first response is to try to assess what we were doing before, and people often return to their previous pattern when they talk about it. As Marj said when people asked her what they'd been doing before, "You want to remember the new thing." The pleaded-for ten minutes buys some time for the new idea to establish. I always promise to answer their questions after this waiting period. Often, however, the questions will have disappeared during the integration time of such an interval.

Ways to Facilitate Turn Taking

A few ideas:

> People write their names on a piece of paper and put them in a hat. As people finish their turns, they pull a paper out of the hat to name the next person. Everyone has the freedom to pass.

> As people arrive, they "sign up" for a turn on a numbered list. I follow the list, always with the proviso that someone can pass.

> If I have a blackboard, whiteboard, or easel, I devote a section of the board for people to write up what they want to do—so, I can simply read requests and questions from the board.

It is the teacher's responsibility to help anyone who may feel reluctant or shy to get the information they need, so I seek ways to help them participate.

Ultimately, you are teaching people that what they want is important.

You Might as Well

At the Friday Harbor Residential, one of the participants noted that she had heard me say several times, "You might as well think of the Alexander Technique." Her omniservation shone a spotlight on how often *you might as well* shows up in my process—I found out that I say it a lot. By the end of the residential, it had become a whole-group refrain.

I remember consciously developing this idea while learning the Alexander Technique. My day job was at a bank. It wasn't what I wanted to do with my life, and I thought I might as well use the Alexander Technique as I did my job. In lines at airports, in the dentist chair, waiting at a checkout line—I might as well play with what I know.

You might as well was part of Marj's teaching process, too. Many a time I heard her say, "This is what you might as well be doing." There is an ease, a lightness to this phrase—a reminder that the Alexander Technique is a little something you can try out from time to time. *You might as well* carries a message of confidence in your ability to do it, as well as the always-needed freedom to choose.

You Never Know What Will Happen from What You Say

Here is the last paragraph of an article I wrote for the issue of *Direction* about kids:

> Parenting can only be learning—our children, our situations are continually changing. And yet, as a parent, perhaps my greatest challenge is to learn to be a parent rather than to try to be a good parent. It is through Alexander's discoveries that I shift my perspective to my moment-to-moment interactions rather than to some imagined end result. If I see parenting as a process of learning about myself and my children rather than something I am supposed to do in some right way, then I think I will be teaching flexibility and coordination to my children—in their bodies, in their minds, and in their hearts. (Madden 1990, p.224)

At the Alexander Technique Congress in Sydney, some time after the article was published, a teacher approached me and said, "You don't know me, but I want to show you a picture." He took out his wallet and shared with me a lovely picture of a baby. He related that he and his wife had been having some difficulties because she wanted a child and he couldn't bring himself to want one—until he read my article.

Wow.

This moment was thrilling, one I will never forget—a reminder to me of my responsibility to the sacred space of teaching.

Chapter 31

THE EVOLUTION OF A TEACHING LIFE

The challenge I posed to myself at the International Congress of Alexander Technique Teachers in Engelberg, "How can I teach in such a way that the Alexander Technique process sustains and—if necessary—restores cooperation with our natural design in service of what we do?" along with the investigative practices I initiated then are woven into the fabric of my daily life—teaching and otherwise. I test the Alexander Technique as I use it—for myself and for others—in the fire of direct application.

The timing of this book has proved interesting because I am currently introducing new vocabulary, hence a new nuance, to my own teaching. Toward the end of writing, I taught a workshop at the Freedom to Act Conference in New York (an annual conference on Acting and the Alexander Technique hosted by the Balance Arts Center). The first thing I did was to change the title of the session: it had been called "Creating Your Character's Psychophysical History" and became "Creating Your Character's Biopsychosocial History." We didn't have a blackboard to write all the elements of Engel's definition of *biopsychosocial*, so we created a kind of living blackboard, with each participant responsible for one element. My participants laughed with me throughout the workshop as I occasionally stumbled while choosing my new word rather than the one I have used for years.

Also new is my acquaintance with Daniel Siegel's work on interpersonal neurobiology—particularly his research and experience regarding the "yes" brain, which I reference later in this chapter.

While my work draws deeply on my nearly 20 years with Marj, my teaching language has evolved significantly from how I learned.

A few of the things I have forsaken were a little tender to lay aside; those ways of saying things had served me well, were perfect as I learned them, and were deemed to need an update. In truth, I believe Marj would be pleased—her language in teaching evolved over the time I studied with her. Her Living Room Étude was all about creating the conditions in which I discovered who I am as a teacher.

We evolve.

When I am introduced to a new idea and am considering it in relationship to teaching the Alexander Technique, I have a three-part litmus test.

First, does the idea contribute to a constructive change in the head–spine relationship as I add it to my process? Most new ideas are simply new information about how humans function. Just as helping someone locate their atlanto-occipital joint benefits their ability to ask themselves to COORDINATE, switching from using *psychophysical* to *biopsychosocial* does not require me to do anything, simply to use the same process with new knowledge. If it helps, great; if it doesn't, also great, but I move on.

Second, does my new idea, or teaching idea, resonate with, or match, or further explicate some aspect of the educational process outlined in "Evolution of a Technique"? Is it an educational process? There are many worthwhile pathways for healing, for developing strength and skill, for spiritual practice—all of which the Alexander Technique could serve; and they, in turn, might serve the Alexander Technique. They are, however, outside the educational umbrella of this work.

Third, is the idea connecting or distracting? When humans find themselves discoordinating in particular circumstances, distracting ourselves is a way to get respite from the interference—we are giving ourselves a break. This may be a step toward what we ultimately want. But, every so often, that step can be mistaken for the solution. It is a little like the odd instruction actors and musicians might get to pretend the audience isn't there. For a moment, a day, this might offer a "Band-Aid" to a particular issue that needs a deeper resolution. It will ultimately fail because it isn't true—the audience is there, and when the performer resolves the actual interference, they become better artists. Any suggestion that avoids, attempts to keep people away or back, or says "no" to the truth of the present moment doesn't pass this third criterion of my litmus test. It may be a needed respite or tactic on the way, but it is a detour from the Alexander Technique and its ultimate use—whole-self withing—the biopsychosocially vivacious presence with self and others—in action—in the world.

Current Report of My State of Evolution

A prominent scholar once called me, wanting lessons to assist with writer's block. He had studied the Alexander Technique in the 1940s in London and thought a renewal might be helpful. At the conclusion of the first lesson, during which we cleared my desk (he christened it "an archaeological dig") so he could use it, he said, "You'll do," and scheduled another session. When I looked at him quizzically, he said that he and his original teacher in London had talked about how you could use the Alexander Technique process to teach anything, so it was important to know what the teacher thought they were teaching. It wasn't that I had specifically stated, "This is what I am teaching." I had taught the lesson as I teach, and it matched how and what he wanted to learn.

Wow. You can use the Alexander Technique process to teach anything, so it is important to be clear about what you are teaching.

Alexander Aesthetics

In the chapter on "Tactile Communication," I talked about the career crisis I had experienced in Engelberg. The teaching ideas offered in this book comprise the ever-evolving report from the research and self-scrutiny renewed that afternoon in the Alps.

What emerged from my initial query of what I dubbed "Alexander Aesthetics"—via studying human coordination and Alexander Technique teaching models in a variety of ways, and questioning and clarifying my own teaching choices—is how lucky I was to have learned the Alexander Technique directly in relationship to doing what I want to do, how lucky to test its efficacy in action I chose and cared about. Direct application ensures that the Alexander Technique is serving life. And while everyone who learns the Alexander Technique needs to learn how to integrate it with their life, direct application makes this considerably easier because the activities we do in classes, lessons, and workshops become external cues, reminding us to use the already-integrated-with-activity studied rehearsed plans to do what we do. Direct application keeps my process honest through its constant feedback from reality-based practice. I believe this is what the scholar with writer's block recognized.

The "Yes" Teaching Perspective

I believe that I have taught the Alexander Technique and coached acting from a "yes" perspective for most, if not all, of my teaching career. While I am convinced this is what I learned in the Living Room Étude, I first christened the term "yes perspective" as I prepared for my sessions at the International Congress in Lugano in 2011. A detailed explanation on why "yes" matters follows, yet it can be understood as simply as the "Don't Think of a Pink Elephant" story. The *only* way not to think of a pink elephant is to think of something else. The "yes" of this new thinking causes thoughts about that irresistible pink elephant to disappear.

Characteristics of My "Yes" Perspective

1. "Yes, I want to use the process to be with whatever I am doing, with whomever I am with," is a yes to engagement with my biopsychosocial world, desiring to respond to stimuli. All Alexander Technique teaching is necessarily tied to some activity, because it is about how you do what you do, rather than an end in itself. By insisting on applying the Alexander Technique teaching only to real things we do, we prevent an inbred aesthetic and insist on practicality. Because all teaching of this work requires something to do, why not do things that are pertinent to each individual—from their first lesson?

2. *Yes* becomes "yes you can," believing that all of us are fully capable of learning this work and applying it on our own, from our first encounter with the process. What I learned from Marj taught me that I needed to say "yes" to myself as a prerequisite for teaching. She always said "yes" to me in some way—whether it was in her first note to me about moving to Nebraska, her "why don't you think about it for a while?" or her "yes" when I asked her if she thought I was ready to teach a course at the University of Nebraska. "This is a great DO IT YOURSELF program. I think I'm teaching in such a way that students are beginning to understand more and more that

they can do it for themselves after a very simple introduction" (Stillwell 1981, p.21; original emphasis).

3. It is my job to teach from this belief for my own students.

4. *Yes* preserves my freedom to choose. *Yes* awakens me to my own volition with abundant possibilities of response. *Yes* opens the dance of creativity because all options are available. *Yes* offers dynamic moment-to-moment sovereignty in my life. If someone in my introductory series tries to restrict their activities because "they couldn't possibly use the Alexander Technique to do them," I say, "If learning the Alexander Technique restricts you from doing anything that is humanly possible, I believe that you should run screaming from the room!"

Choosing "Yes" as the Leading Idea in Teaching the Alexander Technique

My delight at being introduced to Daniel Siegel's work is that his research supplies data supporting the "yes" approach to human development. His most recent book is, in fact, entitled *The Yes Brain: How to Cultivate Courage, Curiosity, and Resilience in Your Child* (Siegel and Bryson 2018). Aren't these qualities we want for ourselves and for our students? Aren't these qualities we hope the Alexander Technique supports? I mentioned Daniel Siegel's yes/no exercise in Chapter 7, "Having a 'Yes' Plan." In further describing his experiential demonstration of the differing responses of groups to hearing an alternating series of spoken "yes" and "no," Siegel says:

> What I think this exercise reveals is our two fundamental states: "no" evokes the reactive state, "yes" evokes the receptive state. Reactivity has its roots in our ancient reptilian past, the 300 million-year-old brainstem being activated with a state of threat that gets you ready for the four fs of fight, flight, freeze, or faint. In contrast, a younger 200-million-year-old mammalian circuit soothes the brainstem's alarm bells, turning on the social engagement system that opens us up by making us receptive. Our muscles relax, we can hear a wider range of sounds, see a wider range of things in front of us. This is the neural correlate of our open, receptive state, ready to connect and learn. (Siegel 2017, p.309)

With the teacher's "yes" at the door of the studio augmented by the "yes" of the learners walking through the door, new capabilities are unveiled. Our quest is the ability to respond wholeheartedly—yes—with our whole selves—yes—to the stimuli of our lives—yes—engaging with each other—yes—and the world—yes—as we do what we need to do—yes—to pursue our highest dreams. Yes.

Alexander Technique International (ATI)

Alexander Technique International is a worldwide professional organization created to promote and advance the work begun by F.M. Alexander. Its members include teachers, students, and friends of the Alexander Technique. I am one of the founding members of Alexander Technique International, have served as its Chair, and have been Chair of the Vision/Mission Committee.

http://www.ati-net.com

Our Mission

1. To create and sustain open means of global communication for people to discuss, apply, research, and experiment with the discoveries of F.M. Alexander.

2. To encourage the use of the F.M. Alexander Technique in both human and environmental relationships.

3. To embody the principles of the F.M. Alexander Technique in ATI's structure and means of operation.

4. To provide a means for recognizing Alexander Technique Teacher competence and providing certification for those teachers who qualify.

Storytellers

Steve Blakeslee
Amanda Cole
Lynne Compton
Diego de Acosta
Anita King
Carol Levin
Ellen Mross
Sherill Roberts
Fia Skye
Crispin Spaeth
Tony Tengs
Debbie Young

References

Ackerman, D. (1999) *Deep Play*. New York: Random House.

Alexander, F.M. (1984[1932]) *The Use of the Self.* 3rd ed. Downey: Centerline Press.

Aristotle (2013) *Poetics*. Translated by A. Kenny. Oxford: Oxford University Press.

Barstow, M. (2009) "Short Introduction to the Alexander Technique by Marjorie Barstow." Accessed on 13/1/2018 at https://www.youtube.com/watch?v=isz5XVqFrFU.

Barstow, M.L. and Brenner, W. (1987) "Practical Marj: Article and Interview." *Direction* 1, 2, pp.28–37.

Berthoz, A. (2000) *The Brain's Sense of Movement*. Translated by G. Weiss. Cambridge, MA: Harvard University Press.

Blakeslee, S. and Blakeslee, M. (2007) *The Body Has a Mind of Its Own: How Body Maps in Your Brain Help You Do (Almost) Everything Better*. New York: Random House.

Boal, A. (2002[1992]) *Games for Actors and Non-Actors*. Translated by A. Jackson. New York: Routledge.

Brown, S. with Vaughan, C. (2009) *Play*. New York: Penguin Books.

Chekhov, M. (1991) *On the Technique of Acting*. New York: HarperCollins.

Clarke, J.I. (1998) *Who, Me Lead a Group?* Seattle, WA: Parenting Press.

Coyle, D. (2009) *The Talent Code: Greatness Isn't Born. It's Grown. Here's How*. New York: Bantam.

Csikszentmihalyi, M. (1996) *Creativity: Flow and the Psychology of Discovery and Invention*. New York: HarperCollins Publishers.

Dewey, J. (1938) *Experience and Education*. New York: Collier Books.

Duhigg, C. (2012) *The Power of Habit: Why We Do What We Do in Life and Business*. New York: Random House Publishing Group.

Durie, B. (2005) "Senses special: Doors of perception." *New Scientist* 2484, p.34.

Dweck, C. (2006) *Mindset: The New Psychology of Success.* New York: Ballantine Books.

Engel, G.L. (1978) "The biopsychosocial model and the education of health professionals." *Annals of the New York Academy of Sciences* 310, pp.169–187.

Ericsson, A. and Pool, R. (2016) *Peak: Secrets from the New Science of Expertise.* New York: Houghton Mifflin Harcourt.

Etymonline.com (2018) *Online Etymology Dictionary.* Accessed on 28/3/18 at http://etymonline.com/word/desire.

Fluegelman, A. (1976) *The New Games Book.* New York: Headlands Press.

Fluegelman, A. (1981) *More New Games.* New York: Headlands Press.

Gallagher, M. (2005) "Creating new neurological pathways to find freedom from post-traumatic stress disorder." *Direction* 3, 4, 24–29.

Gottschall, J. (2012) "Why Storytelling is the Ultimate Weapon." Accessed on 29/11/17 at www.fastcompany.com/1680581/why-storytelling-is-the-ultimate-weapon.

Hagen, U. with Frankel, H. (1973) *Respect for Acting.* New York: Macmillan.

Holmes, N. and Spence, C. (2004) "The body schema and the multisensory representation(s) of peripersonal space." *Cognitive Processing* June 5, 2, 94–105.

Huizinga, J. (1949) *Homo Ludens: A Study of the Play-Element in Culture.* Translated by R.F.C. Hull. London: Routledge and Kegan Paul Limited.

Jones, F.P. (1997) *Freedom to Change.* 3rd ed. London: Mouritz Ltd.

Jory, J. (2000) *Tips: Ideas for Actors.* Lyme: Smith and Kraus, Inc.

King, D. (1964) *Training with the Organization: A Study of Company Policy and Procedures for the Systematic Training of Operators and Supervisors.* London: Tavistock Publications.

Knowles, M., Holton, E., and Swanson, R. (2005[1973]) *The Adult Learner.* 6th ed. San Diego, CA: Elsevier.

Kyle, P. (2012) "100 Days: Peter Kyle Dance." Accessed on 21/12/17 at https://vimeo.com/84650337.

Leonard, K. and Yorton, T. (2015) *Yes, And: How Improvisation Reverses "No, But" Thinking and Improves Creativity and Collaboration.* New York: Harpers Business.

Libet, B. (2004) "Do We Have Free Will?" In B. Libet, A. Freeman, and K. Sutherland (eds) *The Volitional Brain: Towards a Neuroscience of Free Will.* Exeter: Imprint Academic.

Lieff, J. (n.d.) "The Volitional Brain: Towards a Neuroscience of Free Will." Searching for the Mind with Jon Lieff, M.D. Accessed on 22/12/17 at http://jonlieffmd.com/resources/volitional-brain-neuroscience-free-will.

Lieff, J. (2013) "Small Choices That Can Change Your Life in Great Ways." Accessed on 22/12/17 at www.mindbodygreen.com/0-11467/13-small-choices-that-can-change-your-life-in-great-ways.html.

Linden, A. and Perutz, K. (2008) *Mindworks: An Introduction to NLP*. Bethel, CT: Crown House Publishing LLC.

Madden, C. (1990) "A perspective on parenting." *Direction* 1, 6, 221–224.

Madden, C. (2005) "Refurbishing images in actors and others." *Direction* 3, 4, 9–12.

Madden, C. (2012) "Deep play variations." In S. Jones (ed.) *Congress Papers: Learning from Each Other*. London: STAT Books.

Madden, C. (2014) *Integrative Alexander Technique Practice for Performing Artists: Onstage Synergy*. Chicago, IL: University of Chicago Press.

Madden, C. and Juhl, K. (eds) (2017) *Galvanizing Performance*. London: Singing Dragon.

Morris, E. and Hotchkis, J. (2002[1977]) *No Acting Please*. 5th ed. Los Angeles, CA: Ermor Enterprises Publishing.

Palmer, P.J. (1998) *The Courage to Teach*. San Francisco, CA: Jossey-Bass Publishers.

Palmer, P.J. (2000) *Let Your Life Speak*. San Francisco, CA: Jossey-Bass Publishers.

Pert. C.B. (1997) *Molecules of Emotion: The Science Behind Mind–Body Medicine*. New York: Touchstone.

Piper, W. (2002[1930]) *The Little Engine that Could*. New York: Platt & Munk Publishers.

Rickman, A. (2010) "Alan Rickman on Importance of Listening when Acting." BBC News. Accessed on 26/11/2017 at www.youtube.com/watch?v=BfytKK6gyVE.

Rilke, R.M. (1986) *Letters to a Young Poet*. Translated by S. Mitchell. New York: Random House.

Rosen, M. and Oxenbury, H. (1989) *We're Going on a Bear Hunt*. New York: Simon and Schuster.

Sachs, J. (2012) *Winning the Story Wars: Why Those Who Tell—and Live—the Best Stories Will Rule the Future*. Boston, MA: Harvard Business School Publishing.

Schirle, J. (1987) "An Interview with Marjorie Barstow." *a.c.a.t west newsletter* 2, 1, 4–6.

Seyler, A. and Haggard, S. (1946) *The Craft of Comedy*. New York: Theatre Arts Books.

Shakespeare, W. (1974) G.B. Evans (ed.) *The Riverside Shakespeare*. Boston, MA: Houghton and Mifflin Company.

Siegel, D.J. (2012) *Pocket Guide to Interpersonal Neurobiology: An Integrative Handbook of the Mind.* New York: W.W. Norton & Company.

Siegel, D.J. (2017) *Mind: A Journey to the Heart of Being Human.* New York: W.W. Norton & Company.

Siegel, D. and Bryson, T. (2018) *The Yes Brain: How to Cultivate Courage, Curiosity, and Resilience in Your Child.* New York: Bantam.

Stillwell, J.O. (1981) "An interview of Marjorie L. Barstow on the Alexander Technique and its history." *Somatics* 3, 3, 15–21.

University College London Psychology and Language Sciences (2017) "Audience Members' Hearts Beat Together at the Theatre." Accessed on 23/11/17 at www.ucl.ac.uk/pals/pals-news/audience-members-hearts-beat-together.